This Is
Not
Your Father's Body

*Fitness, Health and Nutrition
For Middle-aged Men*

By James Judd, B.A.

National Library of Canada
Cataloguing in Publication Data

Judd, James, 1952-
This is not your father's body : fitness, health and nutrition for middle-aged men
Includes bibliographical references.
ISBN 1-55369-193-8
1. Middle aged men--Health and hygiene. I. Title.
RA777.8.J83 2002   613'.04234   C2002-900267-2

TRAFFORD

This book was published *on-demand* **in cooperation with Trafford Publishing.**
On-demand publishing is a unique process and service of making a book available for retail sale to the public taking advantage of on-demand manufacturing and Internet marketing.
On-demand publishing includes promotions, retail sales, manufacturing, order fulfilment, accounting and collecting royalties on behalf of the author.

Suite 6E, 2333 Government St., Victoria, B.C. V8T 4P4, CANADA

Phone	250-383-6864	Toll-free	1-888-232-4444 (Canada & US)
Fax	250-383-6804	E-mail	sales@trafford.com
Web site	www.trafford.com	TRAFFORD PUBLISHING IS A DIVISION OF TRAFFORD HOLDINGS LTD.	
Trafford Catalogue #02-0006		www.trafford.com/robots/02-0006.html	

10   9   8   7   6   5   4   3

Every physician, including myself, has experience with patients for whom overwork, overeating, daily stress and a lack of basic exercise and nutrition curtails both the quality and quantity of daily life.

This unfortunate situation is worsening rather than improving, especially in view of the post-second-world-war population bulge and an ever-growing group at the middle age and senior years. Health-care systems are overtaxed and we, as individuals must assume some responsibility to assure that whatever level of personal health possible is attained and maintained. We must all be introspective.

This particular book targets a particular aspect of the population (middle-aged men), but I believe it applies equally to all regardless of age or sex. The younger one starts, the easier to maintain oneself. Parents should not only begin themselves, but pass knowledge to their children.

I personally have benefited enormously by initiating and maintaining a lifestyle of exercise and nutrition in recent years.

James Judd is to be congratulated on producing a book of immense value, based on his own experience and personal philosophy. The middle-aged group of men is a reasonable starting point and those agreeing in principle should feel confident that by utilizing an outline such as in this book it is possible to achieve and maintain no matter what age you begin.

Don't hesitate! Begin today!

Dr. Malcolm L. Wilson, MD, FRCS (C),
Diplomat of the American College of Surgeons

Table of Contents

Foreword iii
Introduction 1
Chapter 1: 13
Nutrition - The Key to Life

Chapter 2 48
Foods You Should Never Eat

Chapter 3 56
Free Radicals and Anti-Oxidants

Chapter 4 65
Detoxification

Chapter 5 72
Out of the jungle and into the gym

Chapter 6 83
The Gym Exercises

Chapter 7 104
Free Weights or Machines?

Chapter 9 111
Aerobics And Cardio Conditioning

Chapter 10 115
The Home Gym

Chapter 11 125
Attitude and Self-confidence

Chapter 12 130
Clothing And Gear

Chapter 13 134
Stress And Other Detriments

Chapter 14 144
Personal Appearance And Hygiene

Chapter 15 156
Get Into Your Kitchen

Conclusion 184
Bibliography 189
And Additional Reading

ii

Foreword

There are many people who have provided me with inspiration, support and love during the long tenure necessary to bring this work to fruition. To these individuals I humbly dedicate this book. They include Dianne, for her tireless reading and editing advice, Jonboy, J.J., Doyle, Eddie and Grant in the newsroom.

John, for being such a good friend, Joyce for her devoted support and for Kirby and the kids - Bram, Carson, Cassidy and Christine. And last, but not least, it is for my parents, especially my father. God rest his soul.

It's never too late to be
what we could have been

Introduction

This book contains a lot of information pertaining to health, fitness and the well-being in general of men like you and I. Middle-aged men, that is.

Some of what's written here deals with the science of nutrition, while other areas delve into the specifics of muscle building and body shaping. There is far too much for anyone to learn in one lifetime in any one of these areas, but take from it what you can, add to it what you already know, and from it all become someone and something greater than you already are.

What this book is really about is choices. As if we aren't faced with enough choices throughout our lives, here we are faced with the task of choosing between the road well-travelled and the road seldom taken. By this, I mean you can make the choice of millions of North American men to sit on the couch and stuff yourself with unwholesome food, watch television until your mind is numb and perhaps consider walking to and from your automobile as your daily exercise.

The other choice is to break free from the decadent, easy life and instead take a path that will make you lean, hard, keen and strong - sound of body, sound of mind.

The first choice requires that you likely do nothing you aren't currently doing. The latter will require of you a commitment to yourself. That choice is to eat nutritious food, drink pure water, to work at improving your muscle mass and to preserving your bone density.

The rewards for choosing this way of life include a better, healthier, younger, more sexy body than you might have had at any time previously. It also means a new lease on life - a better quality of living for what could amount to a much longer period of time - perhaps as long as 100 years or more.

There is no guarantee you'll live longer as a result of reading this book or by faithfully following the advice it contains. Alas, a long life is not the natural consequence of eating properly and exercising vigorously. There are too many variables and life tends to be unpredictable, even if we do follow all the rules and try to keep our noses out of trouble. Accidents happen and people are sometimes struck down in the prime of life for no other reason than that they were in the wrong place at the wrong time.

So are you the kind of man this book is targeting? To find out if you might be, read these next few questions and take an objective look at the person in the mirror:

If you are now at mid-life or beyond, how do you measure your success?

A huge bank account? A senior position with a major corporation? A beautiful house? Cars, boats and a lengthy assortment of toys?

But when you look at yourself in the mirror, whom do you see? Does it still look like that wiry, handsome kid who graduated high school or do you see a paunchy, balding, overweight, overstressed middle-aged man?

No matter how much money you make in this life, no matter how many cars you will own, houses you can purchase or dream vacations you can afford, the simple fact is you only get one body. What's more, if you've invested your life in the pursuit of financial wealth - at the expense of your health and fitness - you have missed the boat.

If you aren't now and have never been taking care of yourself - body, mind and spirit - you needn't bother investing dutifully in retirement saving programs. You may as well spend that money pre-paying your funeral arrangements and devote the time shopping for a funeral plot. You are far more likely to need these services than you are likely to require a vast amount of money for a retirement lifestyle because that is going to be a lot shorter and a lot less fulfilling than you ever imagined.

Regardless of how much material wealth you accumulate, what good is it if you haven't got your health? How can you enjoy the best years of your life if you haven't got the energy to get off the couch, the muscle coordination to walk without the aid of a cane? What fun can the outdoors possibly be if you haven't the physical capability to exert yourself once in a while without worrying that you may suffer a heart attack?

On the other hand, if by the time you reach 50 years of age and you still have the physique of a 20-year old, then you have truly accomplished something. Consider yourself a truly wealthy person.

So what age is your body right now and we aren't talking about chronological age. How's your eyesight? What do your biceps look like? How are those triceps? What does your belly look like? Can you still see your feet when you look down?

If you look like the average North American man, the thought of looking objectively at your own body probably makes you wince. So, take comfort in the fact that it's not too late to turn things around - provided you are willing to make the commitment.

Bad habits and gravity may have done a number on your body, but by making some lifestyle changes, it can be redeemed - inside and out. You can rebuild it so it is healthy, robust, strong and lean. This is not fantasy, this is not about cosmetic surgery or implants or anything artificial. This is not only possible, it can actually be achieved in a shorter time than you might have thought.

This book is not about instant cures, but it is definitely a miracle cure if you stay with it and make it part of your lifestyle. Wouldn't you rather spend your 75th birthday or even your 100th birthday rollerblading to the gym for a workout instead of shuffling down to the nursing station in the rest home?

The fact is, if you are like the average middle-aged man in North America, you indulge in too much overprocessed or fast food, too much sugar and simple carbohydrate, too much alcohol, too much fat-laden food, too much snack food and too much of too many other body-killing compounds. There is also likely too much stress in your daily life and you probably know little, if anything, about how to deal affectively with it.

And overeating isn't the only culprit. For most adults, inactivity is as much to blame for being overweight. In fact, inactivity often leads to overeating and a craving for high-carbohydrate, high-fat foods containing little or no nutritional value.

4

The irony of being alive in these times is that the age of communication has never been easier or more accessible. People can be in touch with anyone at any time from almost any location. At the same time, people have become almost completely out of touch with their bodies - they don't know anything about what makes them tick. They simply don't know what they need to nurture and nourish them from the inside out.

If you are one of these individuals, then right now is the time to start making the necessary changes in your life. It's time to live better - healthier, smarter and fitter.

— — — —

Once in a while, whether for reasons of self-assurance, or perhaps just to reaffirm my own smugness, I'll dig out an aging, black-and-white photo of myself perched on my father's knee. It was during my first summer back in 1953.

The most startling feature about my father isn't the period clothing as much as his period features. He was only 32 years of age at the moment that photo was taken, but my Dad looks tired, overweight and out of condition. He had also lost almost all his hair by that point in his life and looks for all the world like he's suffering from a doozy of a hangover. Clearly, he looked burned out and middle-aged at 32.

Later, by the time I was graduating high school and my father had indeed reached mid-life, he was a man sliding hopelessly and inevitably towards old age and so were many of the men of his generation. My own father did live to see mandatory retirement. Unfortunately, like so many others, he didn't go much beyond - expiring many years before he should have. In the end, he was frail, gaunt and almost unrecognizable as the man in those earlier photos.

But the way things turned out wasn't entirely my father's fault. There was far less information about the long-term benefits of proper nutrition, and too little education dedicated to promoting the hazards of such potentially dangerous practices as cigarette smoking. Men of my father s generation gladly lit up unfiltered cigarettes, and smoked dozens of them each day. To make matters worse, they would frequent beer halls, pubs and parlours in which the air was often thick and blue with second-hand smoke.

Ironically, most of those men began life in a cleaner environment than we did, and a much cleaner atmosphere than any subsequent generation will enjoy. As well, they generally ate food that was free of preservatives and additives, much of which might have been organically grown.

In fact, it wasn t until the end of the Second World War that pesticides, herbicides, fungicides, growth hormones, antibiotics and a host of other contaminants began to routinely find their way into our food supply.

So why did the previous generation seem to age more quickly? In short, it was the attitude. Their concept of aging was considerably different than what we now accept. Then, it was generally accepted that at 30 a man s youth was long gone. Middle age was also considered a major turning point in life and it generally arrived long before 50 years. For the most part, the previous generations bought into the theory that the chronic conditions of old age were an inevitable and therefore irresistible consequence of a natural life. Therefore, the course of their lives followed what they believed about aging.

Similarly, if anyone buys into the getting-old-is-inevitable theory, they too are probably well into the act of premature aging. The only difference between how you looked and felt as a young man, and how you look and feel today is the use - or disuse - of your muscles. You need your muscles as much when you are older as you did as a young person - perhaps even more. Without muscle you won t be able to balance properly nor will you be able to perform simple daily tasks. Eventually, you may not be able to lift yourself out of a chair. Maintaining muscle mass will also ensure that your bone density is maintained. In turn, this will prevent many of the degenerative bone diseases and disabilities that are often associated with the aging process.

The baby boom generation is always gathering knowledge so they can stall the onset of aging. We also have an insatiable thirst

6

for a better quality of life. We like to snub our noses at the concept of growing old. So if you aren't happy with the way you look right now, all you really need is the desire to look better because the technology and the equipment is available to make this happen. Repeat this to yourself:

I want to look better

I want to feel better

I want to be better

I want to do it now!

With plenty of role models presenting a different face of aging, the boomer generation refuses to go quietly into middle age and certainly won't be any happier to slide quietly into their golden years. If possible, most of us intend to take our youth to the grave. Some of us may even succeed. In truth, everyone knows you can't take your wealth or your health with you, but which would you rather have just in case they're wrong?

One of my inspirational idols is a man named Henry Caulker. Henry is a former Canadian and world champion bodybuilder. Although he no longer competes, Henry remains one of the most sought-after guest posers at bodybuilding competitions. He maintains a low body-fat index, has plenty of muscle mass and more cuts (high muscle definition) than you'd believe possible. But the most surprising thing about Henry isn't his excellent physique; it's the fact that he was born in 1936. His appearance is stunning and, coupled with the fact that Henry is a true gentleman, he is certainly a great role model for men of any age. Henry has also been featured in a number of bodybuilding and muscle magazines.

On any given day, Henry can be found working out with a couple of partners, both of whom are young enough to be his grandsons. They pay a lot of attention to the advice Henry hands out, because they hope to look just like him one day. They can only hope they'll still look like him in another 40 years.

So where does this idea come from that age takes away our strength? How often have you heard people try to justify their lack of strength, or their sedentary existence, by saying, "It's my age?" Henry is just one example that this does not have to be the case. What's more, there are people far older than Henry who are still power lifters and body builders - some even into their 80s and beyond.

Another example is Jack Lelanne, who is now heading towards 90 years of age, but is still one of the fittest men on the planet. Not one of the fittest senior citizens, mind you, but simply one of the fittest men. His feats of strength would be considered incredible even if he were a very young man. He's not a freak of nature; he has just dedicated his life to staying in tremendous physical condition. He has proven that muscle power will stand the test of time, but it makes him seem very unusual by comparison to men his age.

The cases of Lelanne and Caulker aside, it has been proven in a number of case studies that weight-bearing exercises can have positive muscle-building results on people even in their 80s and 90s. It's never too late, but the earlier you get started, the better off you'll be.

Anyone can look good in their 20s, but to look young and lean and have well-defined muscle mass well into the later years - the 40s, 50s, 60s and beyond - requires a much different philosophy, not to mention a lot more discipline and desire. Men like Henry Caulker and Jack LeLanne look terrific at their age. But the truth is, they look good for any age!

— — — —

Education continues to be the key to slowing the aging process. The more you know, the further you go (and the more youthful you'll grow?). We have an ever-increasing volume of work on the subjects of fitness, health and nutrition. Having a good all-round knowledge of these areas enables just about anyone to live a healthy, vibrant life and to remain strong and vital.

Canadian author and nutrition expert Sam Graci, who published an outstanding book called The Power of Superfoods, said this about the process of aging:

"After a quarter century of nutritional research, I have concluded that progressive deterioration can be slowed, and that the human body can operate efficiently in a youthful state well into our nineties or maybe even to 120.

Today, anti-aging researchers agree that many of the symptoms we associated as biomarkers of aging - wrinkled skin, memory loss, hearing difficulties, lack of vigor and energy, cancer, arthritis, weight gain, osteoporosis, degenerative disease, lack of enthusiasm, hair loss, loss of lean muscle mass and strength - may be more associated with improper nutrition than chronological aging."

Eating properly, getting plenty of rest, and exercising regularly doesn't have to consume your life, nor cost a lot of money. On the contrary, eating organic, wholesome food and drinking good, clean water can be cheaper than the way you're probably living right now.

While it's true we have a lot of advantages our fathers never had, it goes a lot further and a lot deeper than advancements in science, technology, and communication. Most of our fathers didn't have a gym around the corner. They didn't have power foods and wholesome food concentrates that can make the job of building muscle easier, faster and more efficient. When our father's bodies began to break down, they ran for the doctors. Well this is not your father's body. If you don't like the body you have, you can do something about it, starting right now.

And don't be anxious if you are already past 50, or even 60 or 70. There's no reason to believe good health and a more youthful body can't be achieved at any time. Starting later only means you may have to work a little harder, and that you may also have to drop a few more bad eating habits. You're only too old to change if you think you're too old. Don't be afraid to adopt new attitudes and to try something new.

Much of the problem is what we are currently eating which includes a diet high in processed and refined foods that are essentially devoid of nutrients. This kind of eating only serves to starve our bodies of the precious nutrition it needs for growth and maintenance. If any components of good nutrition are compromised, metabolic function will be impaired, opening the door for weight gain and for toxins to accumulate.

Thanks, but no thanks, Dad

From an early age, I knew I didn't want to be like my father. He was the butt of jokes for my friends, who enjoyed kidding me about my dad's pot belly, or his bald head, or the way he was "feeling good" all the time, or the number of times he was carrying beer into the house instead of groceries. It hurt me to think a grown man could be such a joke while many of my friends' fathers were still young and healthy-looking. My philosophy, from very early times, was to somehow survive to a ripe old age, while maintaining a youthful and vital appearance.

That began a lifetime of collecting information on the aging process . . . a gathering of information on proper diet, nutrition, weight training, mental health, and emotional well-being. These were the tools I would need if I was to arrive at middle age and beyond with my youth intact. They are the same tools you will need.

I did arrive at some dead ends, made many mistakes along the way, and tried things that didn't work. Eventually, I was able to create a physical presence that has for a long time been a trademark of my life. I have achieved lasting muscle mass and muscle tone, and am blessed with extraordinary vascularity, good circulation, and healthy, resilient skin. When people think of me - at least the ones who know me - they immediately get a mental image of health, because this is who I am to these people.

With 50 just round the corner, I feel I've achieved what I set out to do so long ago. Along the way I've counselled hundreds of individuals, advising them on some of the best ways to achieve, and maintain, a healthy and vital lifestyle. This information has not only helped them turn back the clock, but has also prepared them for the long road that lies ahead. That may not mean living to be 100, but it will mean a better quality of life along the way. It will also ensure they will enjoy doing the things they've always enjoyed, and will enable them to have the energy and vitality to take on new challenges along the way.

Long ago I made a promise to myself that I would struggle to look better at 30 than I did at 20, better at 40 than at 30, better at 50 than at 40, and so on. I easily met my goal at 30, and just as easily met my goal at 40. Now, as the last days of my 40th decade are coming to a close, my body continues to respond to the physical challenges I throw at it. Not only have I been able to maintain the muscle mass and shape that I had worked to achieve for decades, but I'm actually beginning to look better as I approach 50 years of age.

But there's much more to the big picture than simply looking good. The key is to become healthy - inside and out - and to maintain that high level of health. This is absolutely essential in these times, as health care deteriorates and health care budgets continue to be slashed.

Now, more than ever, prevention is the name of the game, and that means finding the best, most healthful diet possible. It also means starting a weight-lifting program

For some, this will mean they need only to fine-tune their diet and/or exercise regimes, while others will take a look in the mirror for the first time in a long time and wonder where they will start to undo the years of abuse and neglect.

If you are among the latter, have faith and believe that you can indeed undo the bad and make it good again. Some may need more time than others, but be confident that you too can become healthy, fit and shapely in a half a year or less.

There are no quick fixes here - no corners to be cut, no miracle machines to do the work for you. It requires a lifetime of commitment to a new and better lifestyle.

On the other hand, waiting just on the other side is a long, rich fulfilling life of well-being, health and oodles of energy and vitality. It makes everything better - from your attitude about yourself, to your confidence levels, to your sex drive.

When I first stepped into a gymnasium almost 30 years ago, the variety and availability of quality supplements was extremely limited. These were also difficult to find, unless you were living in Southern California, or in a huge metropolitan area. Protein powders were available, but weren't nearly as sophisticated as they are now. Much had yet to be learned about the processes that now enable these supplements to be efficiently used by our bodies in the process of building muscle and reducing fat. There have been huge advancements in other supplemental areas such as the introduction of creatine and glutamine - two wonderful products that can aid anyone in building lean muscle mass while ridding themselves of body fat. Remember that for every additional pound of body fat, the blood must be pumped through an extra mile of blood vessels and capillaries. How much do you think are you overtaxing your own heart right now?

There has also been a carbohydrate revolution taking place in recent decades. Complex carbohydrates - the kind that sustain energy over long periods - can be easily consumed in liquid and solid form with plenty of good taste to go along with the nutritional benefits.

But there's also plenty of good, old-fashioned sweat equity that has to go into building and maintaining a better body. Without discipline, hard work and patience you could simply crash and burn along the way. Keep in mind that there is no finish line in the road of life.

12

Chapter 1:
Nutrition - The Key to Life

If you are the average North American male, you likely spend more time taking care of your automobile than you do caring for and nurturing your own body. Too many North American men ignored their nutrition lessons while growing up, preferring to ingest knowledge of things mechanical. You probably relied on your mother to keep you healthy and nutritionally fit.

Unfortunately, the physiological changes that take place between adolescence and adulthood, especially for men, are such that there is a sudden and dramatic falling off of testosterone production. This not only lowers our sex drive, but also changes a great many other things, including the way we metabolize our food. The result is a tendency to accumulate fat at the expense of lean muscle mass. This is accelerated in later years as we turn to a more sedentary lifestyle - laying on a couch, watching sports on television, and snacking on high-fat, processed foods. Add to this the accumulated affects of over-processed fast foods, too much sugar, too much alcohol, too much smoking; too much of everything that doesn't agree with us physically, but which tends to satisfy us emotionally.

Following this type of lifestyle is certain to get you just one place - six feet under! Even if it doesn't kill you outright, you're on a collision course with a heart condition, a stroke, or possibly both. This means you'll eventually end your days in a nursing home, where you'll spend your time worrying if you're getting enough medication or enough care, or possibly why your family doesn't want to come and visit.

Okay, that's not painting a very pretty picture, but there's no point in sugarcoating the truth. If you are currently abusing your body with bad food, bad water, and bad habits, this is what comes of it.

But eating and living properly is going to require some immediate changes. Rest assured these changes are essential for your health and well-being, as well as for obtaining and maintaining maximum fitness and physique levels.

As adults, we've been conditioned to believe the dieting concept that has been around for as long as there have been people concerned about their weight. Chances are, you've followed the North American trend, and have been on at least four diets already during your life. But diets are little more than a Band-Aid solution to a much bigger and more complex problem. Diets don't do anything for nutrition, but are generally tied to deprivation and craving. Eating the right kind of foods, in the right balance, on a daily basis, will take away the necessity for weight-loss diets.

What we're going to cover here are the fundamentally important ingredients for every good body. They are fats, carbohydrates, protein, vitamins, fibre, soya lecithin and water.

This is an oversimplified concept of good eating and healthy living, but if you understand the basics, you can easily apply a much broader application. Once you grasp the fundamentals of good nutrition, you'll be able to guide yourself through the rest of your years. From here, you can expand your knowledge and your experience in order to get the most out of your body, your mind and your remaining years.

Learn to enjoy food for its healthful benefits, not to fear it, or to be enslaved by it.

Fat

Fat is one of the key ingredients for good health and well-being. Too much of the wrong kind is deadly, while getting enough of the right kind is not just essential, but instrumental in building and maintaining your body from the inside out.

By now, you might be asking yourself the questions, "Good fat?" "Bad fat?" What on earth can this mean?

We all consume fat on a daily basis, but most North Americans ingest a steady diet of the deadly, rancid, hydrogenated variety. Fast food, fried food and the like, as well as potato chips, nacho chips, chocolate, and a host of other items we consume regularly, are essentially killing us. While these fats do contain Omega 6 essential fatty acids - something necessary to our bodies - they also contain something called trans-fatty acids. These serve mostly to raise cholesterol levels and cause degeneration within our organs.

Trans-fatty acids, like those in margarine and other hydrogenated oils, along with heavy metals, alcohol, and other chemicals and drugs, add to the breakdown of our arteries, which then need to be repaired. Unfortunately, when the artery is weakened, cholesterol and other proteins are used to make repairs, resulting in a thickening and hardening of the arterial walls.

Avoiding toxins like trans-fatty acids, and consuming poly-unsaturated fats like those found in flax seed, fish, and sunflower oils, also help reverse the condition known as atherosclerosis or hardening of the arteries. These essential fatty acids make the arterial walls stronger and more flexible.

A little less than 70 per cent of people in North America die each year from just three conditions, all of which are brought on by fatty degeneration. These are:

cardiovascular disease, which accounts for more than 43 per cent of deaths in industrialized nations;

various cancers - which account for a further 22+ per cent of deaths;

and diabetes, which accounts for less than two per cent of deaths.

Changing the type of fat we eat, and staying away from the kind of fat we have been eating, will help us in a big hurry.

What our bodies really need are Omega 3 fatty acids, in balance with those Omega 6 fatty acids mentioned earlier. The combination of these essential fatty acids creates a kind of harmony within our bodies that is difficult to describe, in terms of its positive effect. The positive changes are almost miraculous, almost as soon as we begin getting proper amounts of these essential fatty acids. They play key roles in the construction and maintenance of all healthy cells.

The fats we are promoting for good health are obtained from pure, raw food sources. These oils must come from raw, unprocessed seeds, nuts and vegetables, which were once abundant in the food we ate. But these have become scarce since the arrival of overprocessing, and heat-treating food and oils for esthetic purposes and convenience of consumption.

Our bodies use unsaturated and essential fatty acids to construct membranes, create electrical potentials, and move electric currents. It can also burn them to produce energy if the vital roles these fatty acids play have been adequately filled. To make a long story short, if we are ingesting good fatty acids on a daily basis, our body is getting what it needs, and will begin burning stored fat as an energy source. This means we actually get leaner by eating fat. It is a paradox, but it works.

The best sources of these essential oils and fats are raw nuts and seeds, such as flax seed, sunflowers, pumpkin, walnuts, pecans, almonds, hemp seeds, soybeans and soy nuts, and a host of others.

Fortunately, we can easily ingest all the essential oils we need every day by simply purchasing any number of specially prepared oils currently available. Somebody has already done all the work, while taking the guesswork out of balancing the Omega 3 and 6. The best of these are Udo's Choice, and another known as Essential Balance. In addition, a number of good quality hemp seed oils are also available, which naturally combine a balance of Omega 3 and Omega 6 essential fatty acids.

These essential oil compounds combine Omega 3 and Omega 6 fatty acids derived from organically grown, cold-pressed nuts and seeds like flax, pumpkin, sunflower, borage and sesame, as well as wheat germ oil and a few other carefully-selected ingredients.

Consuming these essential oils on a daily basis will have a profound and lasting affect on your body, your energy levels, and your general well-being. They help each of the body's internal organs to function properly, and chief among these is the way it helps to regulate the production of insulin in the pancreas. This, in turn, helps to smooth out energy levels, and to prevent cravings for simple carbohydrates and sugars during the course of the day.

Other benefits will be noticed quickly as well. For instance, many lingering maladies such as sore joints, tendonitis, and the like usually disappear, and the skin will take on a smoother appearance, and will regain much of the elasticity and resilience that it has lost over the years.

In an effort to find these essential fatty acids that it craves, your body has been programmed to store all the fat you've been consuming, so that it can find the right kinds of fat it wants and needs. Once you begin ingesting the right kind of essential fat on a daily basis, your body will begin burning off the old, stored fat as energy, as it begins a process of house cleaning.

The overall effect is a much happier liver, too. Since our livers must process the fats and oils we eat, ingesting the right kind on a regular basis, while cutting out or at least cutting back on the bad types, will have an immediate, profound, and lasting effect on this organ.

What's more, essential fatty acids are utilized by the most active tissues of our body, such as the brain, sense organs, adrenal glands, and testes. Again, ingesting the proper fats, on a daily basis, means proper functioning of all these key areas.

Incidentally, another good source of essential fatty acids are green, leafy vegetables, so a healthy salad every day, with a dressing made of essential oil, apple cider vinegar, and a few herbs is not only delicious, but nutritious and satisfying as well.

This is only a simplified version of the story behind good and bad fats. It does cover the basics, however. But if you require a more complete explanation, and I highly recommend that you seek further information on this topic, refer to the book, "Fats that Heal, Fats that Kill," by Udo Erasmus. It was first published in 1986 under the title Fats and Oils.

Udo Erasmus has earned international recognition as an authority on the subject of good and bad fats. He actually pioneered the technology for pressing and packaging healthy oils.

When you go looking for your source of essential oils, go directly to your local health food store, where you'll find them stored in refrigeration units. Once you purchase these, store them in your refrigerator and use them within a few weeks, to prevent them from going rancid. Essential oils are very fragile in comparison to those manufactured through heat processing and they can't be subjected to heat or light, or the nutrients will begin to deteriorate.

They must also be consumed in their raw state, and never used for cooking. If you must cook with anything, use oils such as butter, canola, grape seed, or olive oil, which remain intact at higher temperatures.

For the time being, and if at all possible, avoid frying anything, however.

Apple Cider Vinegar

This compound, made by fermenting fresh-pressed apples, is one of the true power foods when it comes to daily nutrition and overall wellness. With the exception of apple cider vinegar, all other vinegars should be avoided, since they contain a destructive ingredient known as acetic acid.

Pure apple cider vinegar, on the other hand, made from whole apples and not diluted, contains a constructive ingredient known as malic acid, which is an ingredient, needed in the digestive process. The malic acid found in this vinegar - which tastes delicious when used in salad dressing, by the way - combines with alkaline elements and minerals in the body to produce energy, or to be stored as glycogen for future use.

There are a lot of benefits derived from using apple cider vinegar on a daily basis. It will virtually clear up any and all skin irritations. It will also help kick-start your metabolism, and thereby help maintain the liptrophic, or "fat-burning," process that we are striving for. But the most outstanding property of this wonderful supplement is that it will balance the acid-alkaline levels in your blood, giving it the proper PH level it needs to keep you healthy and strong.

When you are working out, and your muscles begin to lactate at the end of a set of repetitions, drinking a little apple cider vinegar diluted with water will very quickly restore your strength, by helping to normalize the PH of the blood getting to those muscles. As a result, you should be able to recover more quickly and be ready to go just as hard on the next set. If you don't mind the taste, mix a few tablespoons into your water bottle and sip it continually while you are working out. You'll notice a big difference in your energy levels over the course of the workout.

Again, this product is available at any health food store, but is also available at some of the larger food chain shopping centres. Be careful not to get "flavoured" vinegar, which is essentially just white vinegar with apple flavouring and colour added.

What you want is pure, raw, unfiltered, unpasteurized apple cider vinegar. Be sure to read the label if you're not certain about the ingredients.

Take at least two tablespoons of this wonderful stuff every day. Some people simply pour it onto a tablespoon and take two of these, followed by a drink of water to wash it down and dilute the taste. You can also add two tablespoonsful to a glass of water and drink this.

Another way to ingest it is to make a salad dressing, by combining equal parts of apple cider vinegar and essential oil. You can use an essential oil blend for this, or you can use straight flax seed oil, which on its own is the richest source of Omega 3 essential fatty acids. After combining the two ingredients, give it a taste test. If it's a little bland, try seasoning it with Mrs. Dash, or with a ready-made product called Spike. The latter is a wonderful combination of sea salt and some 30-odd herbs and spices. This product is also available in health food stores, as well as many grocery chains.

You can experiment with the amount of Spike or Mrs. Dash until you find a likable dressing you can pour on your salad once or twice each day.

Incidentally, apple cider vinegar also works as a powerful analgesic, so if you have sore muscles, try rubbing it on the area and massaging it in. Within a few minutes you'll feel plenty of heat, just like you would if you had used an analgesic balm.

It works by drawing blood to the surface of the area on which it has been applied. Knowing this, some people have rubbed it on their thinning and balding scalps, and have reported varying degrees of success in regenerating their receding hairlines. If you want to give it a try, do so before you go to bed, however, since it can smell a little strong.

Taking apple cider vinegar will also do wonders for your circulatory system. If you've been having circulation problems, they'll clear up in short order as you dose yourself each morning with this wonderful super food.

This substance also works topically as a remedy for varicose veins. Many women and a good number of men, particularly those in middle-age, suffer from this affliction. Diluting apple cider vinegar one-to-one with purified water, and applying it directly to the affected area, will bring surprising results.

Carbohydrates

In a nutshell, carbohydrates come in two basic forms - simple and complex. We need a little of the former, and quite a lot of the latter, in order to function properly, and to have the energy our muscles need to perform. However, we North Americans tend to overeat from the simple carbohydrate group - sugar and sugar-laden foods - and tend to get less than we need from the complex group, which includes fruits, vegetables, whole grains and legumes (beans), peas, sprouts, and grasses.

When we eat foods that contain these complex carbohydrates, the digestive tract easily breaks them down into glucose, which is then transported, via the blood, to wherever it is needed in the body as energy, whether it's the muscles, the internal organs, or the brain. What isn't used is stored by the body as glycogen for future use. Glycogen only occurs in the body, not in any food, and is the reserve of glucose stored by the body in the muscles and in the liver for future use.

The glycogen stored in the muscles is used as glucose for energy whenever we indulge in some activity, whether it's working out in the gym, swimming, dancing, or running to catch an elevator. Meanwhile, the glycogen stored in the liver is used as an energy source for the internal organs, as well as the brain.

How you are able to perform at any of these physical tasks, including your daily workout, depends on how much glycogen is stored in your muscles. Too little means you will suffer from early fatigue; but that also triggers the production of a pancreatic secretion which turns stored fat into glucose, which can then be used as an energy source. As you can see, this bodes well if you are trying to reduce your body fat level through a program of weight training combined with aerobic activity.

However, the downside to this is that once the glycogen stores have been depleted, the brain triggers another mechanism whereby muscle is broken down into glucose, which is then used as an energy source. So, it's a fine line between getting lean and getting emaciated if you don't eat properly.

To maintain a good store of glycogen in the body, we need to consume a good amount of complex carbohydrate each day - as much as 50 or 60 per cent of our caloric intake, in fact. However, because complex carbs are good for us, people mistakenly believe they can eat as much as they want. Like everything else, too much of a good thing will do you harm.

When we eat carbohydrates, our blood sugar level (the amount of simple carbohydrates floating around in the blood supply at any one time) rises, and the pancreas responds by secreting insulin. This is a hormone designed to restore blood sugar equilibrium within our bodies. It does this by removing excess glucose from the bloodstream, which is then stored as glycogen in the liver and muscles. However, what can't be stored there, is then stored as fat.

Now you can see the connection between simple sugars and fat storage, right? In spite of the fact that a container of designer frozen yogurt claims to be fat-free, it is still loaded with sugar, and those simple carbohydrates are stored quickly as fat. Every time you down a half litre or so of a soft drink from a convenience store, or slurp one of those gigantic frozen slushes, you are putting unwanted fat into your body, especially if your body already has all the glycogen stores it can use.

The bottom line here is that if you are consuming huge quantities of sugar on a daily basis - donuts, cakes, cookies, ice-cream, pastries, etc., etc. - you can be almost certain that they are being stored as fat.

Now you can more clearly understand that the misconception that eating fat will make you fat, isn't necessarily true.

Worse still, high insulin levels in your body will block the release of fat-burning glucagon. How many times have you seen somebody running on a treadmill, or riding a stationary bike, or working out on a stairmaster while sipping a soft drink at the same time? It makes the whole exercise a waste of time, if they are attempting to burn fat, because their bodies are getting a fresh supply of carbs to burn, therefore eliminating the need for the body to break into its glycogen stores.

So, how much complex carbohydrate does one need in the course of a day? Well, there is a simple formula to determine this amount, and from this we simply determine how much food is necessary in order to achieve the desired amount of carbo intake.

Since we ideally should ingest 55 or 60 per cent of our daily diet intake as complex carbohydrates, this means a daily caloric intake of 2,200 calories - about the amount an average-sized man would require - should be about 1,200 to 1,300 calories from complex carbohydrate.

Since each gram of carbohydrate is comprised of about four calories in food value, we then divide 1,200 by 4 and arrive at roughly 300 grams of complex carbohydrate each day.

The best choices you can make, as far as sources for these complex carbos, are fresh, preferably organically grown, fruits, vegetables, whole grains, beans, sprouts and leafy greens. A word of caution in regards to potatoes and rice, though. Potatoes have a surprisingly high glycemic index, as does almost all varieties of rice, with the exception of whole-grain, brown rice. A high glycemic index simply means the carbohydrate in the food is broken down quickly and sent directly into the blood stream. So, potatoes and rice are better as an after-workout meal, rather than before a workout.

All sugars are not simple carbohydrates either. White sugar, or sucrose, as well as brown sugar, syrup, honey and most other sugars, are broken down quickly. However, fruit sugar, or fructose, is broken down quite slowly - about one-quarter the speed of white sugar or honey. This may seem odd, or even out of character, but these are the facts.

And, as strange as it may seem, many fruits are broken down slowly in the body, while others put their simple carbs into the bloodstream very quickly. Cherries and pears have a low glycemic index. Apples are moderate, while bananas are very high. Again, the former could be eaten prior to a workout, to supply extra energy, while the latter can be eaten afterwards to replace depleted stores of glucose.

For more information on this subject, you might want to refer to some of the new books on the market which deal specifically with the glycemic index.

Another good idea is to have plenty of colour variety when it comes to these fruits and vegetables . . . yellow, orange, green, red, etc. The more colours, the better. If you consult a standard food chart or carbohydrate counter booklet, it will give you a good idea of how much carbohydrate is in each of these foods, which should then make it relatively simple to consume the right portions.

When choosing your carbohydrates, choose the least processed varieties you can find, and your preference should always be for organically grown. For instance, choose organic, brown rice over processed white; whole-grain hot cereals over boxed, processed variety; an apple over an apple fritter or turnover; an orange over frozen orange juice concentrate, and so on.

Avoid processed convenience foods, which are made with refined white flour and hidden sugars, and are almost certain to contain hydrogenated vegetable oils and other trans-fatty acids. Try reducing your consumption of refined grains such as white bread, white pasta, and white rice, which are essentially devoid of nutrients.

As far as bread goes, the best choices are either those made with organic, sprouted grains, such as pumpernickel or rye bread -

preferably the dark variety. These latter two breads will help to maintain a high metabolic rate, and can actually help you reduce your fat stores over time. However, don't mistakenly run out and start eating nothing but rye and pumpernickel breads in an effort to lose weight and/or fat stores more quickly. A slice or two a day, along with the other complex carbohydrates, is more than enough.

Just before we go any further, it should be pointed out that meals should be consumed more often during the course of the day. If you've been used to the usual three squares a day, do some rethinking now. A better solution is to break up your daily caloric intake into six or seven small meals, which should be eaten two and a half to three hours apart throughout the day. This type of eating helps to keep your metabolic rate at a premium. What's more, it will also prevent hungry periods, when you may be inclined to stuff something less than desirable into your mouth in order to satisfy your hunger.

The best solution is to have a big breakfast, then pack a mid-morning snack, preferably a high-protein, high carbo one. Then, have a decent lunch and pack another mid-afternoon snack. Have a decent dinner - not too large, then another mid-evening snack, each time carefully including lots of protein, some complex carbohydrate, and some dietary fibre in the mix.

Protein

Protein is one of the most important foods we need on a daily basis. As much as a fifth of a person's total body weight is protein and next to water, it is the most plentiful substance in the human body. Without protein, our bodies could not produce or store energy, and we need the nitrogen found in protein to build and repair body tissue, like muscle.

What you probably don't know about protein is that we don't get it directly from the foods we eat - even if they are comprised mostly of protein. Instead, our bodies break down the foods we eat into amino acids, from which they build their own protein. To accomplish this, our bodies require 22 amino acids - all but eight of which it can synthesize on its own. These eight include: isoleucrine, leucine, lysine, methionine, phenylalanine, valine, tryptophan and threonine. Don't worry, you don't have to memorize these names, and there's not going to be a test at the end of the book.

However, in order for the body to manufacture its own protein, all eight of these essential amino acids must be available at the same time. Foods which contain all eight in the proper abundance, and in the proper proportions for human development, are the best proteins available. These include powdered egg whites (egg albumin), hydrolyzed, lactose-free whey protein, and soy protein isolate powders.

The next group of foods that can be used as a rich protein source include fish, free-range eggs, skinless poultry - particularly chicken breasts - and lean meats. The third-best food group is the low-fat and non-fat dairy products.

At the bottom of the list are seeds, nuts, legumes, sea vegetables, bee pollen, whole grains, and nutritional yeast.

Protein helps slow the rate of entry of carbohydrates into the bloodstream, thereby maintaining a steady amount of insulin secreted by the pancreas, and thereby assuring a steady energy source.

The amount of protein we need on a daily basis has been the subject of controversy for a number of years. However, there is no rule of thumb that covers everyone. Some people can get by on less, but others, particularly those who are working out in a gymnasium, need a lot more. You will be among this latter group, so pay attention.

For our purposes, let's say you will need to consume between three-quarters and one gram of high-quality protein per day, for each pound of body weight. That means if you tip the scales at 180 pounds, you will require between 135 and 180 grams of protein daily.

What's more, protein intake must be spread out over the course of the day, in order to be properly utilized by the body. At one sitting, the body cannot synthesize more than about 30 grams of protein. Therefore, it becomes necessary to eat five or six meals each day, with each meal supplying approximately 30 grams of good-quality protein.

A lot of people will consume huge amounts of red meat at one sitting, or may get most of their daily protein intake from meats with a high fat content. Try to get your protein intake from protein supplement powders, whole egg whites or powdered egg whites, skinless chicken breasts, or fresh and canned fish.

Whenever possible, buy meats and poultry from sources that offer animals bred and raised free of antibiotics and/or growth hormones. Remember that these, too, are ingested, and stored in the muscle tissues.

Protein must be chewed thoroughly, to aid in the process of digestion, so that you get all the benefit possible from what you are eating. This is a non-negotiable command - chew your food thoroughly!

By chewing each mouthful 25-30 times - I know, that seems like a lot - the chewing process breaks down the food while saliva is mixed with it to initiate the digestion process. If you eat hurriedly, failing to chew more than five or six times, you will end up passing much of the beneficial elements through your digestive tract. The good stuff will come out the other end, and only the easily digestible elements will remain in the system. It's inefficient and will slow your progress greatly, leading to frustration when you are looking for positive results.

This chewing business applies not only to solid food, but also to your high-protein shakes, drinks and snack bars. Chew even your protein drinks before swallowing, to mix saliva and get the digestion working in the mouth. Otherwise, you simply won't benefit as much as you should from what you are eating, and you'll be wasting protein and other nutrients.

Speaking of protein shakes, plan to have at least two each day, in addition to the meals you will be consuming, in order to get your daily intake of protein. It isn't the protein itself that is creating the muscle, remember, but the process of breaking muscle cells through weight resistance, then rebuilding them with the protein manufactured by your body.

Mix your shakes in a blender, and add your essential oil at this time, which makes it much more palatable for some. Others won't mind the taste of the oil, which tastes somewhat like melted butter and is very nutty-flavoured. Nevertheless, if you have a problem getting it down, put it in the shakes. Also, add a tablespoon of soya lecithin powder. As a base, try using fresh fruit juice such as unpasteurized, unfiltered apple juice, or freshly squeezed orange juice. If neither of these is available, get used to using purified water as a base.

You can use milk as a base, but it isn't recommended. Filtered whey protein doesn't mix well with milk, and besides, many adults are either lactose intolerant, or may simply have an allergy to bovine milk. It can create gas and bloating in those who have an intolerance to the sugar found in milk (lactose).

Another option for the protein shakes is fresh fruit, such as strawberries and/or bananas, or even fresh pineapple. It adds good carbs and additional fibre, as well as more living enzymes.

There are many convenient forms of protein supplementation on the market these days, including protein bars. However, be aware that many of these bars are mostly sugar and simple carbohydrate, in addition to the protein they offer. If you shop around, you can find some bars now that offer high-quality protein and almost no carbohydrates at all; these are preferable, though costly. In fact, protein bars are perhaps the least cost-efficient source of protein available, though they are perhaps the most convenient.

However, we are trying to get away from the convenience of eating, and into trying to enjoy what you eat while making it work efficiently for you. Still, if you find you need the convenience occasionally, go ahead and buy the protein bars.

It is possible to build a good muscular physique on a vegetarian diet - even a vegan diet. It was once thought that vegetarians had to eat foods in combinations at each meal, in order to complete the protein chains and thus allow the body to produce its own amino acids.

However, now it has been found that if you eat various types of legumes, nuts and seeds throughout the day, your body's protein pool can combine various plant proteins gathered during the day to achieve its full amino acid quota. This type of diet can provide plenty of protein if it's drawn from a wide variety of sources. You'll still want to supplement this kind of eating with high-protein drinks, however.

Lecithin

A substance found in all cells of the body, lecithin is a fatty acid that prevents cell membranes from hardening. It is most prominent in the brain, heart, liver and kidneys.

Lecithin is composed primarily of choline and inositol, which are necessary for the breakdown of fats and cholesterol. Lecithin breaks up the cholesterol so that it can be transported easily through the blood without clogging arteries, which, in turn, lessens the chance of heart disease.

The choline component is also a necessary compound for neurotransmissions, governing actions such as memory, mood, and muscle control.

It is thought to reduce the risk of liver degeneration by aiding fat metabolism in that organ. It also facilitates the absorption of vitamin A, vitamin D, and thiamine in the intestine. It is also effective at reducing nervousness and as a treatment for depression. Taking a daily lecithin supplement can also reverse skin irritations such as eczema and dermatitis.

The body can manufacture lecithin from foods such as whole eggs, but the cholesterol level of whole eggs becomes somewhat prohibitive as a source for manufacturing this substance. Therefore, the best way to supplement your diet with lecithin is to simply purchase it in granular form from your nearest health food store. It is inexpensive and easy to consume, since it tastes nutty and dissolves with relative ease in blender drinks. You'll need to ingest one or two tablespoons each day over a period of time to notice the effect.

There are some interesting and beneficial side affects to taking a lecithin supplement, as well. It has been known to increase sexual prowess, and is also beneficial for increasing the volume of ejaculate in men. If you think this won't do something for you, as well as your love life, think again.

Fibre

Your goal should be 35 to 50 grams of fibre as part of your daily diet. This is more than double the average North American daily fibre intake of 15 grams or less. Mostly, this inadequacy is due to the overprocessing of foods and the lack of good fibre in most fast-food diets.

If you aren't currently getting 35 to 50 grams of fibre daily, be aware that you don't want to rush out and stock up on high-fibre foods and fibre supplements to correct the problem overnight. Your body doesn't like that much change in that brief a period, and you'll end up with some severe bowel problems if you attempt this.

Rather, gradually increase your fibre intake, along with your water intake, since fibre absorbs water and creates large, soft stools that move through your bowel easily and, are passed quickly and easily, too.

Don't stock up on one type of fibre either - such as oat bran, wheat bran, or corn bran, and especially not psyllium husks. And don't rush out and buy a case of Metamusil, either. There are seven basic fibre types including bran, fruit pectin, mucilages, cellulose, gum, lignin and hemicellulose, The body needs a combination of all of these in order to make your bowels function properly and regularly, since each type has a unique function.

Research indicates that a high-fibre diet will help prevent blood clots, colon cancer, and varicose veins, but it also stabilizes blood sugar levels by slowing the release of sugars from digesting foods, which is vital if you hope to reduce body fat levels. It also works to remove toxins and heavy metals from the body.

By eating a diet that includes foods which contain these basic fibres, you'll enjoy peak performance. These foods include whole grains, nuts, beans, flax seed, hemp seed, pumpkin seeds and sea vegetables.

Spread your fibre intake over the course of the day, trying for an ideal level of eight to 10 grams per meal over five or six meals.

In addition to the seven basic types of fibre, these are also broken down into two groups: soluble and insoluble. Many foods - such as legumes, fruits and vegetables - contain both types.

Insoluble fibre promotes more efficient elimination and leads to a reduction of colon cancer and intestinal disease. Brown rice, wheat bran, vegetables, legumes and the skins of fruits and vegetables are excellent sources of insoluble fibre.

Soluble fibre lowers blood cholesterol by grabbing hold of it and ushering it out of the body. Good sources of this type include oat bran, apples, prunes, grapefruit and legumes.

Vitamins, Minerals and Supplements

Iron: Because only a small amount of iron in the foods we eat is actually absorbed by the body, we need to either eat substantially more iron-rich foods daily, or take a daily iron supplement, or a vitamin supplement containing the mineral.

The iron from animal foods - called heme iron - is more readily absorbed than is the iron from vegetable sources - nonheme iron. In fact, about 23 per cent of the iron in meats, fish and poultry is absorbed, while only about eight per cent from vegetable sources - including dark greens, fruit, grains, legumes and eggs - is absorbed.

An iron deficiency can lead to anemia, which causes that light-headed feeling people often get after exerting themselves at some activity. Anemia is a condition in which our blood contains insufficient hemoglobin, the part of the blood that transports oxygen from the lungs to the tissues.

It should be noted that vitamin C is an iron enhancer. Taking a vitamin C supplement, along with an iron supplement, or drinking a glass of orange juice or carrot juice with an iron supplement, will enhance the absorption by the body.

On the other hand, tea and coffee are iron inhibitors. Drinking either of them with iron-rich foods, or taking an iron supplement with them, will inhibit its absorption.

Some other iron-rich food sources include blackstrap molasses, green leafy vegetables such as broccoli and bok choy, organ meats, and eggs.

Vitamin C: Vitamin C is necessary for the manufacture of collagen and elastin, chemicals that keep arteries, bones, skin and all other tissues strong. Without enough vitamin C to strengthen the tissues, arteries become weakened, and the body uses cholesterol to repair the arterial damage, resulting in thickened, hardened arteries.

Vitamin C can also boost the body's immune system, and prevents unwanted bacteria and parasites from invading the digestive tract. It also has antiviral, antibacterial and anti-cancer properties.

More importantly, it also increases intracellular gluthione and T-cell action. T-cells are a specialty type of white blood cell which fight infection, viruses, and bacteria that get inside the cells of our bodies.

The recommended daily dosage is very low, so be sure and get at least 500 mg per day, but 1,000 mg is even better. Some bodybuilders take as much as 5,000 or 6,000 mg daily, along with their other supplements because it's thought to reduce swelling, aid in the healing of muscle injuries, and to ease joint pain.

There are a few important points to remember about vitamin C, particularly if you are taking heavy daily doses. For one thing, it is an acid and will serve to unbalance your acid/alkaline balance (this is covered later).

The acid can also crystallize and collect in joints, resulting in soreness and stiffness of the joints, much like a mild case of arthritis. In large amounts, it can also be hard on the kidneys, and you may notice frequent urination if taking large amounts. This is a sign that you are getting an over abundance of the vitamin, or that you should be taking a buffered variety.

Buffered vitamin C is a safer and easier way to get a good source daily, since buffering with calcium helps slow the dissipation of vitamin C in the body. Buffered varieties are also easier on the entire system, so if you plan to increase your daily dosage, be certain to take the buffered kind. It is more expensive, but worth the extra money.

Zinc: This is one of the most important mineral supplements a man can take. Zinc regulates the hormone that converts testosterone to the troublesome DHT (dihydrotestosterone), which is the male hormone metabolite linked with excessive prostate tissue growth.

Zinc also helps promote healing, and is essential for healthy hair growth and lustre. It's also an important immune mineral, since it increases the size of the thymus gland, the conductor of the immune system. Without a healthy thymus gland, the immune system is powerless.

Unfortunately, zinc is also one of those supplements where more is not better. Too large a daily dose can be toxic, so never take doses higher than 60 mg per day for prolonged periods. Personally, I find that a 25 mg tablet daily more than does the trick, though I may double that if I come down with a rare cold or flu bug.

Multi-vitamin: Taking a multi-vitamin daily might prove unnecessary if you're already following the dietary program outlined here, especially if you are supplementing your caloric intake with fresh juice. However, any multi-vitamin you take should include beta-carotene and vitamins A, E, and C, along with a B-complex. This combination will ensure you are getting an additional healthy anti-oxidant dose on a daily basis. GNC, a supplement company that has an abundance of outlets in both Canada and the United States, makes one of the best daily vitamin/mineral supplemental tablets. Their product is known as Mega Men. It includes time-release vitamins and minerals, and taking one of these each day should more than suffice your requirements.

Green tea: A source of potent phytochemicals (cell-protecting chemicals) that help to prevent heart disease and cancer, as well as lower cholesterol levels. It is also a powerful antioxidant. Organic, Japanese-grown green teas are the preferred source. However, there are many varieties currently on the market, including some types which include ginseng, Echinacea, and some other herbs. They are all excellent, and extremely beneficial to your general health and well-being.

Trace Minerals: In addition to a number of vital minerals considered essential for human nutrition - calcium, phosphorous, iron, potassium, selenium and magnesium - many minerals are also needed in small amounts to maintain optimum health and well-being.

Although they are often played down, or are largely ignored in the grand scheme of things, vitamins cannot function without trace minerals. These trace minerals also play a role in regulating hormones, enzymes, amino acids and the immune system. They are also required to build and maintain the structure of the body and to maintain proper brain function, blood sugar balance and to help the brain function properly. They are involved in virtually every aspect of health and balance within the human body.

Boron is a trace mineral that helps retard bone loss. It also works in conjunction with calcium, magnesium and vitamin D to help prevent osteoporosis (brittle bones). Boron is abundant in pears, apples and grapes and is also found in raw nuts, green leafy vegetables and legumes such as soybeans.

Chromium is another important trace mineral which works with insulin in the metabolism of sugar, and helps the body utilize proteins and fats. Taken in conjunction with vigorous exercise, chromium also helps the body burn off fat more efficiently. Chromium can also help prevent and lower high blood pressure, and is best taken in the form of chromium picolinate.

Copper works in balance with zinc in the body, and a deficiency of one can result in an overabundance of the other. Copper is essential in order for iron to be utilized, and is also necessary in the prevention of anemia. It's also an important partner with vitamin C in the synthesis of collagen. An excess can also cause hair loss, insomnia, and depression.

Iodine, found in seaweed, seafood, and most table salt, is necessary for proper growth while promoting healthy hair, nails, skin and teeth.

Selenium is another of the trace minerals that is absolutely essential to good health on a daily basis, and men seem to need more of it than women, because it is found in high concentrations in semen. A deficiency can cause dandruff, dry skin, and fatigue, and may be associated with the development of cataracts. Selenium also helps keep youthful elasticity in your tissues, and helps in the prevention of dandruff.

If you're already past the age of 50, it's recommended that you supplement your diet with up to 200 micrograms (mcg) of selenium daily.

Juicing

The best reason I can think of for incorporating fresh fruit and vegetable juice into your diet is the enzyme factor. Raw food, particularly juices made from fresh, organically grown fruits and vegetables, are teeming with living enzymes which the body desperately needs in order to break down the food we eat and to digest it properly and be able to absorb it into our bloodstreams.

Unfortunately, these precious enzymes are extremely sensitive to temperatures. At 120 degrees Fahrenheit, they become sluggish, but at a temperature of only 130 degrees Fahrenheit they die.

Of course, one might wonder why we don't get the enzymes we need simply by eating these fruits and vegetables. To a certain extent we do. However, once we separate the enzymes and the organic water from the fruit and vegetable fibres, this juice is very quickly digested and assimilated - often in a matter of minutes, with a minimum of effort and exertion on the digestive system.

Vital, organic calcium is one of the minerals needed by our entire system and such calcium, which is the only kind that is water-soluble, is only available from fresh fruit and vegetable juices. As such, it passes through the liver and is completely assimilated in the process of gland functions, as well as cell and tissue building.

Gallstones, kidney stones, and gravel in the gall bladder and kidneys, are the natural result of the body's inability to eliminate inorganic calcium deposits formed by eating concentrated starches and sugars.

Within the fibres of whole fruits and vegetables are atoms and molecules which are the essential nutritional elements we require. It is these atoms and molecules, and their respective enzymes, which aid the speedy nourishment of the cells and tissues, glands, organs and every part of our body. Juices extracted from fresh, raw fruits and vegetables are the means by which we can furnish all the cells and tissues of the body with the elements and the nutritional enzymes they need, in the manner they can be most readily digested and assimilated.

Chief among these is carrot juice, which is made by juicing raw, organically grown carrots through a home juicer. These days there are plenty of juice bars springing up, so if you don't mind paying a premium price for something you can make at home for half a buck a glass, do indulge yourself at one of these outlets.

Anyway, carrot juice has the effect of helping to normalize the entire system, and is the richest source of vitamin A; it also contains vitamins such as B, C, D, E, G, and K. It helps to promote the appetite, and is an excellent aid to digestion; it is also a valuable aid in the improvement and maintenance of the bone structures of the teeth.

If you have trouble with your eyesight, and very few middle-aged men don't, drinking carrot juice daily for a period of three or four weeks may do wonders for even the worst conditions of near and farsightedness.

Having indulged in this delightful concoction for many years, I can tell you that I am the only member of my immediate family who has never had to wear eyeglasses. In fact, in the past two years I have had my eyes tested twice, and even as I approach 50 years of age, I still don't require even the weakest prescription for eyeglasses.

The optometrist who has performed these past two examinations has been amazed to note that, unlike other men my age, I can not only read the bottom line of the eye chart with either or both eyes, but I can also read from a book held only inches from my nose.

Nevertheless, your eyesight, should it be failing you, can rebound quickly with daily doses of delicious carrot juice, since it nourishes the optic system.

Carrot juice is also an excellent detoxifier for the liver, giving a wholesale house-cleaning almost as soon as you begin drinking it. In fact, the cleaning of the liver can be so sudden and so complete that the dissolved material, which was clogging it, may be in too large an amount for either the urinary or intestinal tracts to adequately channel through the body. As a result, it is passed into the lymph for elimination from the body by means of the pores of the skin. This material has a distinctly orange or yellow pigment, and while it is being eliminated from the body will sometimes discolour the skin and give it an orange appearance.

It is for this reason that people incorrectly assume that drinking carrot juice, or even eating too many carrots, will turn you orange. It isn't the carrot juice itself that causes this discolouration, however. What it does mean is that your liver was in sad need of a cleaning, and you should be thankful if this does happen, because all it means is that you are now much healthier.

Carrot juice is rich in vital organic elements such as phosphorus, sulphur, silicon, and chlorine, and is a good supplier of calcium, magnesium, and iron, along with alkaline elements like sodium and potassium.

Adding a handful or two of fresh, organic spinach leaves to your carrot juice beefs it up considerably, adding more iron as well as benefiting the entire digestive tract including stomach, duodenum, and small intestine, as well as large intestine or colon.

If you are currently taking some form of over-the-counter relief for constipation, toss it in the garbage and get yourself a juicer. With a combination of carrot and spinach juice or, if you can tolerate the strong taste, spinach juice alone, you'll be relieved of constipation in short order.

Besides, those anti-constipation medications contain inorganic purgatives and chemical stimulants to make the colon expel them. After a while you must begin to take stronger and stronger laxatives since the body adjusts to these irritants. The result is not a cure for constipation, just more and more difficult cases of constipation. On the other hand, raw spinach juice will effectively clean out your bowel, while at the same time healing the bowel and the intestinal tract - something laxatives won't be able to do.

Spinach is one vegetable that should never be eaten cooked. The reason is that cooked spinach contains a high level of oxalic acid crystals, which will accumulate in your kidneys and eventually form stones. If you're one of the unfortunate men who has ever had the misfortune of passing a kidney stone, you'll know the kind of pain and terror that goes on. Therefore, you'll want to avoid the possibility of this ever happening by eating only raw spinach, preferably in juice form.

If, by some circumstance, you are already plagued by kidney stones, don't give them another thought. A combination of carrot and spinach juice will break these up quickly, as will taking either fresh-squeezed lemon juice in water, or diluted apple cider vinegar. Each of these remedies works relatively quickly to dissolve these crystals, and they can then be passed easily and painlessly in your urine.

Juicing raw, organic beets is an excellent way of building up the red blood corpuscles, and toning up the blood in general. One beet, combined with eight to 10 carrots, will provide plenty of juice for this purpose. Again, beet juice is a powerful liver cleanser as well, and this process can occur so rapidly after consuming the juice that it may make you feel a little (or a lot) uncomfortable for a few minutes. This feeling will quickly pass, but if you experience this kind of sensation, once again it's because your liver is in dire need of a good housecleaning.

Juicing green papaya fruit, along with carrots, will provide a juice which will aid digestion greatly, because of the papain enzyme in the papaya. What's more, this combination will work quickly to relieve stomach, intestinal, and duodenal ulcers.

Green, unripe papaya has much more active papain enzymes than does the ripe variety, since for some reason this enzyme dissipates with the ripening process.

Parsley, which is an herb and not a vegetable, is an excellent addition to carrot juice, particularly if you are having trouble with your eyesight. It is effective in dealing with every ailment connected with the eyes and optic nerve system, including weak eyesight, cataracts, conjunctivitis, and laziness of the pupils.

However, never drink it alone or in huge quantities mixed with carrot juice. All that's needed is a small handful to be effective. Too much parsley juice can adversely affect the nervous system.

Another benefit of parsley, whether juiced or eaten in salads or by itself, is that it will sweeten your breath more effectively than any commercial brand of breath mints or breath fresheners.

Herbs

An herb is any plant that has medicinal or healing qualities, though they can also be used as food, and as flavour additives and seasonings. Although in North America we rely mainly on the prescription drug industry as our primary source of healing, almost 80 per cent of the world relies in some way on herbal remedies as its primary care source.

Nevertheless, as much as 40 per cent of prescription drugs are either based on herbal medicines, or are synthesized versions of the healing qualities of natural substances.

Following is a list of some of the more useful and more common varieties which you could begin working into your diet on an occasional basis:

Garlic: It has been said that the ancient Egyptians fed garlic to their slaves to give them more vitality and energy, and to keep them healthier. It has also been noted that at one time the slaves nearly revolted when their daily garlic ration was about to be cut.

Most North Americans think of garlic as flavouring for cooking, or something to be avoided for fear of getting unsociable bad breath. In fact, garlic is truly one of the cheapest and easiest to acquire "wonder drugs." Its use has been well documented throughout history for its antifungal and antibiotic uses. The Russian army used it in place of real antibiotics so often that it was commonly referred to as "Russian penicillin."

The same component that gives the herb its pungent aroma and unsavoury flavour is the one that destroys or inhibits bacteria and fungi. This component is known as allicin, and when a garlic clove is crushed, this component combines with an enzyme known as allinase to offer an antibacterial action equivalent to one per cent penicillin.

Garlic is also something of a tumour inhibitor, and may have cancer-inhibiting qualities. Just remember that cooking garlic diminishes its potency, however. A good habit to get into is eating raw cloves of garlic each night before going to bed. To do this with a minimum of discomfort, chop the clove finely with a large knife, place it on a teaspoon, and swallow it with a drink of fresh water. By doing this, you will hardly taste the garlic, and there will be minimal smell exuding from your pores the following day.

Taken in this fashion, the chopped garlic works its way through your digestive tract during the night, cleansing and helping to get rid of putrid matter, which will be expelled quite easily the following morning. This process will also boost your immune system, and help ward off any cold or flu virus that may be invading your body.

Ginger: Ginger root is another herb that is common and easy to obtain, yet has so many good qualities that it should become a staple in your refrigerator. It is a mild stimulant, promoting good circulation, and can help lower cholesterol levels. It can also prevent blood clotting.

Making a tea of fresh ginger root works wonders for a cold or flu since it is very effective in getting rid of nausea. It is also effective in maintaining a good, high metabolic rate.

Bilberry: Bilberry is also known as European blueberry, and works to improve visual accuracy in healthy humans. However, it is said to also help those with eye diseases such as pigmentosa, retinitis, glaucoma and myopia. It helps anything to do with the ocular area by improving microcirculation, but the active component in the berries is flavenoids, which stimulate the release of vasodilators. These flavenoids are substances which help open up blood vessels, thereby improving the flow of blood, which, in turn, increases the oxygen level in the tissues.

Ginkgo biloba: This is another plant that is rich in flavenoids and which can improve the circulation, thereby addressing problems related to such disorders.

Ginkgo is also effective as a free radical scavenger and has antioxidant properties as well, and these can help slow the processes responsible for premature aging and cancer.

Saw palmetto: This plant has been long used for its ability to improve the condition of the prostate gland and the urinary tract. It is also believed that taking saw palmetto will stimulate and increase bladder contractions, thereby making urine flow easier and less painfully if you are suffering from an enlarged prostate. It can also help to make urination less frequent during the night - a problem that is quite common in middle-aged men.

Aloe Vera: In a liquid form, Aloe Vera is the milky sap found within the fronds of the spiky aloe plant, which has been used for centuries to heal burns. There is nothing better for sunburn than to apply a thick coat of aloe and gently rub it in.

Aloe can also be used as a treatment for stomach and duodenal ulcers, ringworms and shingles. It can be taken orally, full-strength right from the bottle. It is readily available at all health food stores.

Water

Nothing is more important to your body than water. The human body is comprised of roughly 75 percent water, though some areas - the brain, for instance - is comprised of an even greater percentage than the muscles. As we age, this percentage begins the slowly decrease until, as adults, women are about 60 to 62 per cent water and men roughly 65 to 67 per cent. However, as seniors we begin to have our thirst sensation leave us so we become gradually even more dehydrated with age. Water regulates all bodily function and once depleted these function steadily decline.

Without food, human beings can last as long as two months. Without water, it's only a matter of days - two or three, in fact - before we are dead. Water also enables the body to eliminate toxins naturally.

The key to a better, more healthy lifestyle is to begin drinking more water on a daily basis - and we aren't talking about tap water, either. No matter what part of North America you reside in, or what the local authorities have to say about the quality of water coming out of your kitchen taps, drinking city water is a sure-fire way to destroy good health, not improve it.

If you have been existing on tap water for a period of time, or perhaps your life to this point, the water you should immediately begin drinking is distilled water. You can purchase this in quantity, or in personal-sized bottles at any number of locations. If for some reason you simply can't find it, make your own by purchasing a water-distilling unit, if necessary.

The reason for drinking distilled water is that it will help to leach out the toxins and heavy metals that have accumulated in your body over the years. Distilled water is most like organic water in that it can be assimilated into the cells of your body faster than ordinary purified water. Tap water is generally heavily fortified with chemicals and additives to kill bacteria, and to enhance its nutritional affect on your body. However, the liver and/or kidneys must filter out all these additives -some of which are highly toxic - before it is of any use to the body. Be good to yourself and give your filtering organs a break by drinking purified or distilled water from now on.

After you've drunk only distilled water for a week or two, change to purified water and drink only this type for the remainder of your natural life. Again, purified water can be obtained in any number of ways, but the most cost-efficient is to have a system installed in your home. By doing this, you can produce water that is purified by a process of either charcoal filtration or reverse osmosis. Either method will remove the chemicals and contaminants, which actively contribute to the deterioration of your good health.

Water can also help to curb the appetite. In fact, a hungry feeling may be the body's first call for water, but is often misinterpreted as food-hunger. If you are frustrated in your attempts to normalize your body weight and are prone to overeating, particularly in the evenings, try drinking a large glass of water whenever you are hungry, and you may find you no longer desire food.

In some instances, water may contain natural additives that can actually benefit human health. For instance, it's a little-known fact that the people who inhabit the Pacific island of Okinawa routinely live long, healthful lives - many for as much as 110 years. The secret has been traced back to the island's water supplies, which contain high levels of natural calcium gleaned from the minerals and corals from which the island was originally formed. Calcium is a highly beneficial mineral that few North Americans get enough of in their regular diet. Ponce de Leon thought he had indeed discovered the "fountain of youth" in Florida 500 years ago, possibly because the longevity of the natives in the region was based on the same kind of water.

Nevertheless, tap water generally contains harmful contaminants. Chief among these is chlorine - a substance commonly added to urban drinking water in an effort to kill harmful bacteria. While chlorine is effective at accomplishing this, it is also a toxic substance, which can bind with other natural substances in the body to form even more toxic compounds. The result can be failure of various organs to perform their daily functions. In addition, ingesting chlorine can sometimes cause some forms of cancer and/or toxic shock.

Even if you are currently drinking purified water, free of chlorine, it may not be enough to avoid the toxic effects of chlorine. Showering, bathing, and even washing your clothing in chlorinated water can be as bad as drinking it. Your body can still absorb the chemical from the water through your skin and other delicate membranes. If you think for any reason you may be suffering toxic shock, or if you exhibit the symptoms of chlorine poisoning, you might want to look at installing a large enough water filtration system in your home to accommodate bathing, showering, and even washing your clothing.

In addition to its role as a coolant inside the human body, water also lubricates joints, muscles and ligaments. It is important to consciously drink water throughout the course of the day, even if you don't feel thirsty. The feeling of being parched and in need of a drink means your body is already partially dehydrated and you should have topped up your tank hours ago.

Water is also important to the health and elasticity of the skin, both the dermis - the second layer - as well as the epidermis, which is the portion we see on the outside. Dehydration is one of the major causes of wrinkling, and long periods of dehydration will eventually result in irreversible wrinkling.

If you are physically active, be sure to take on plenty of water beforehand, and to consume an adequate amount throughout the exercise period. It is possible to lose up to four kilograms of sweat per hour during an intensive sporting event, so if you are an avid tennis player, a roller-hockey player, or a beach volleyball enthusiast, remember to compensate for the heavy demand for water placed on your body.

If you are in a business that requires a lot of flying, remember that airline flights can also have a serious dehydrating effect on your body. Again, drink plenty of water before your flight, and consume a fair amount during the flight, as well. It will not only keep you fresher and healthier, but you'll arrive at your destination in a better frame of mind, and with clearer thinking. It could prove to be the edge in a deal one day, so take heed.

Even under normal circumstances, you lose as much as six, eight-ounce glasses of water naturally each day. However, excess salt consumption, high climatic temperatures, strenuous activity, intense exercise, and drinking caffeinated beverages such as coffee, tea or soft drinks cause you to lose even more water. Also, dry climates draw out more water from you than do humid ones.

Consuming caffeinated and alcoholic beverages also alters your fluid needs. Caffeine, which acts as a diuretic, increases urine production and also stimulates kidney action. Alcohol inhibits the production of an anti diuretic hormone called vasopressin, which is secreted by the brain.

Drinking a glass of purified water with your morning coffee will help compensate for this effect, while drinking several glasses of water after consuming an alcoholic beverage will also help replenish lost fluids.

Whenever possible, choose purified or distilled water or herbal teas over high-carbohydrate (insulin-raising) sodas, juices, coffee and alcohol.

Reward Yourself

All work and no play is never a way to make people happy and content, so occasionally feel free to eat any kind of meal you want. If you want to sit down to a big plate of lasagna with garlic bread, and have spumoni ice cream for desert, go ahead and indulge.

Not everyone would advocate this kind of binging, but often it comes down to a difficult situation - you are dining out, either at a friend's house or at a restaurant - you may be visiting your parents' place, or whatever. As long as it's no more often than once a week, do feel free to eat any meal you desire. Just be prepared to go right back to the new lifestyle immediately afterward.

Of course, if you become obsessed with only putting good things into your body, but still would like to indulge in something unbelievably rich and tasty from time to time, there is hope. Health food stores also carry a line of organic ice creams, which make even the designer variety pale by comparison. You can also choose to eat frozen yoghurts instead of ice cream.

If you want to avoid all that, but still enjoy desert occasionally, try fruit desert alternatives like organic apple crisp, low-fat cheesecake - made with organic ingredients. Just be moderate about the size of the serving, and try not to make it a habit more often than once or twice a week.

Time Your Eating Properly

Chances are, you're going to be eating more than you were previously, or at least you may think you are. This might create a feeling of uneasiness, or even panic among some. However, eating is going to take place over the course of the entire day, as opposed to stuffing yourself once or twice and going hungry the rest of the time. The latter is how many people ingest their caloric intake each day, and it's nothing more than a recipe for disaster.

Our bodies react differently at different times of the day. They have a high metabolic rate and low fat-storing capacity earlier in the day, which wanes as the day moves on, until evening, which is a prime fat-storing period. A man who starves himself all day at the office, eats a large dinner, then snacks all evening, is going to add inches to his waistline and pounds of stored fat to his body. By adding fat, we also add miles of additional blood vessels and capillaries, through which the heart must pump the blood.

Another thing you'll want to do is throw away your bathroom scales. How much you weigh is no measure of how fit or fat you may be. You can weigh more and still look better, because muscle is denser and therefore heavier than fat. Don't even be tempted to step on the scales once in a while out of curiosity, because seeing your weight will only trigger an older, misconceived notion about weight. You may end up cutting out certain foods you think are making you heavy, but which really aren't.

By following the advice here you will eventually reach an ideal weight. What's more, by that time you'll be fit and muscular, and you won't care about how much you weigh any more.

It's true that breakfast is one of the most important meals of the day, but so are the other five or six you'll be eating. Nevertheless, the metabolic rate and catabolic activity of the body is at a peak at this time of the day, and your fat-storing capacity is at its lowest. That doesn't mean you should sit down to a plate of fried bacon and eggs and a half a loaf of buttered toast, however. Having a bowl of oatmeal or oat bran, half a dozen egg whites, a glass of freshly squeezed fruit or vegetable juice, and a cup of green tea or black coffee will give you six or seven hundred calories with about 30 per cent fat.

Your mid-morning snack (yes, you will be having one of these each day from now on) - around 10 a.m. - should be about 350-400 calories and have a slightly lower fat content - say 25 per cent - even though your body's metabolic rate is still on the high end, and your fat-storage capacity is still quite low. A fruit juice or water-based power protein drink - with essential oil, soy lecithin granules and protein powder - would be ideal at this time.

For lunch, around 1 p.m., you'll want to take in another six or seven hundred calories, but now you cut the fat intake to about 20 per cent of the total calories in that meal. A chicken breast, brown rice with salsa on top, and an organic green salad with a dressing of flax seed oil and apple cider vinegar would do nicely.

The metabolic rate by this time of the day is beginning to drop off, and your fat-storage capacity is moderate now, so by focusing on high-quality protein and complex carbs, we are giving our bodies the best possible combination of foods at this time.

Like mid-morning, mid-afternoon will involve another snack on a daily basis. Once again, the metabolic rate now is only moderate, but you'll want to maximize the free-testosterone levels during your workout later, and this process comes from ingesting fat. The excess fat you ingest now will be used as fuel during the workout, which decreases the storage potential.

Another protein drink, with essential oil and lecithin granules added, would work fine, and would provide the 30 per cent fat that you'll need.

After work, you'll want to work out, so your next meal will be a post-workout snack of about 400 calories, with a low-fat content of 10-15 per cent. This is the time to focus on replacing glycogen stores and moving proteins into muscle cells. More fat now would just slow the absorption time of these nutrients, and compromise your recovery time.

A high-protein, low fat drink would work fine - perhaps just protein powder in fruit juice or water.

An hour or so later, eat dinner, which should consist of six or seven hundred calories, with 20-25 per cent fat. This is the trickiest time, because you want to increase free-testosterone levels to help offset evening metabolism. However, this is also a prime fat-storing time for your body, so a moderate to low-fat intake is recommended.

A meal consisting of a baked sweet potato, broiled skinless, boneless, chicken breast, an organic green salad with the flax seed oil, apple cider vinegar and a cup of green tea, will do the trick nicely.

Chapter 2
Foods You Should Never Eat

Sometimes the battle is lost because guys simply can't give up their favourite high-fat, low-nutrition comfort foods. Worse still, they are eating one or more meals each day from a fast-food establishment, where their lunch or dinner is comprised of mostly saturated fat and empty calories.

Making a lifestyle change means giving up some of the things we cherish. Get used to life without the following killers and you'll be healthier, slimmer, and fitter, just by permanently excluding these from your life:

Mayonnaise: This is one of the most common condiments found in North American households and owing to this fact, it's small wonder the general health of the population is in the state it is. This garbage, particularly the commercial variety, is made of rancid cooking oil which is then partly hydrogenated - meaning they whip air into it to make it firm. The result is toxic goo that is largely responsible for many of the diseases and conditions which relate to poor circulation, free-radical aging, and macular degeneration. And whoever said this stuff tasted good anyway?

Alternatives: None I can think of, or even want to. However, if you must replace this toxic sludge with something, try non-fat, plain yoghourt instead. It has about the same consistency as mayonnaise, but is actually good for your health. You can also try making your own, substituting organic, cold-pressed flax seed or olive oil for the rancid cooking oil, and using egg yolks from either organic or free-range chickens - fresh eggs, not ones ready for the landfill, as in commercial mayonnaise.

Margarine: Like mayonnaise, a toxic substance comprised of hydrogenated, mostly rancid cooking oil. It is as beneficial to your health as used motor oil, and almost as tasty. There are no good brands, no healthy alternatives. This stuff was invented as a replacement for butter, which was in short supply during the war years. Somehow it gained a foothold on the kitchen tables of the world, and the result is almost as many types of cancer as there are types of margarine.

Alternatives: How about butter? In spite of what margarine producers would have us believe, there is nothing unhealthy about eating good, old-fashioned butter, as long as it's used in moderation. Try the unsalted variety, and use butter made from organic milk if at all possible.

Bacon: Filled with chemicals, nitrites and all manner of carcinogenic ingredients, not to mention the fact that it has an extremely high fat content, and is almost devoid of nutrition. Sure, it tastes good, but so does cyanide if you mix it with Kool-Aid, so what's the point? It elevates blood pressure thanks to the high sodium content, elevates bad cholesterol levels thanks to the high fat content, and elevates your chances of getting a number of different cancers due to just about every other ingredient in this hog-belly product.

Alternatives: Flavoured soy bacon-bits, which are available in most supermarkets, as well as health food stores. These still contain a few ingredients on the barely acceptable list, but are much healthier in the long run.

Poutine: It's a big mystery where this recipe for disaster first appeared, but in eastern regions of North America, people line up to indulge in a bucket of this crud. It consists of greasy french-fried potatoes, smothered in gravy, then covered in cheese curds. Your arteries would have a better chance of staying clean if you were to suck the contents of a grease trap through a straw. This is a coronary bypass special if there ever was one. Eating just one order could result in heart failure, a stroke, or even a heart attack. The same goes for eating french fries with gravy. There, you've been warned.

Alternatives: Skydiving without a parachute will get you just as dead as a diet of this sludge. Mind you, it would at least be mercifully quick, and wouldn't end up costing taxpayers the medical bills for people who indulge in this kind of snack. Besides, your body would be less of a mess when it comes time to bury you.

50

Hot dogs: For a lot of North Americans, these are a dietary staple. Each time you consume one of these, you're ingesting 13 to 20 grams of saturated fat, not to mention the same nitrites, toxic chemicals, and high sodium content found in bacon and most other processed meats and meat byproducts. Meanwhile, the processed white flour used to make the roll, along with the high sugar and sodium content of the ketchup, mustard, and other toppings, help make this one of the unhealthiest snacks going. Most schools serve these for lunch to our children, though they are much better prepared to process the ingredients in their digestive systems than are we. Want to add more injury? Try one of the hot dogs filled with process cheese, or even ones filled with process cheese and bacon.

Alternatives: Soy dogs are a meatless alternative to what amounts to basically a meatless product anyway. The European wieners have no preservatives, but are still made with meat byproducts, most of which have been swept off the floors of the meat processing plants, much like their American counterparts. The same goes for similar products like smokies. All have a high fat content, and they all have high levels of sodium.

Processed meat products: Pepperoni, salami, bologna, chicken loaf, mock chicken loaf, etc., etc., etc. Like hot dogs, these are made with meat and meat byproducts that are pressed together with extreme pressure and heat. They all contain plenty of fat and high sodium levels, not to mention high levels of carcinogenic nitrites, chemicals, and other toxic debris.

Alternatives: You don't need any of this stuff in a healthy diet, and there's really no point in trying to find any replacements. Get used to living without this sort of thing.

Fish and chips: If you ever want to know how not to eat properly, visit Great Britain some time. Whatever nutritional value was in the fish to begin with is completely lost after it is coated in a batter of pasteurized milk and processed flour, then deep-fried in rancid grease that contains a high level of saturated fat and trans-fatty acids. Ditto for the chips. You can ingest enough saturated fat to give yourself a coronary or a stroke with just one serving. You'd be better off to discard the fish and chips and eat the newspaper its wrapped in. - you'll do less harm to your body, and you'll likely get as much nutrition. Avoid also fish burgers and other deep-fried, breaded fish products served on white rolls - with rancid sauces, to make matters worse.

Alternatives: Fresh fish such as salmon or halibut, sprinkled with herbs and baked or broiled, served with lemon wedges, a fresh green salad and either a baked potato or organic brown rice and a little salsa on top.

Frozen pizzas: If you could possibly heap as many chemically laced, toxic, nutrient-dead ingredients as possible into one product, it would be called frozen pizza. In addition to being filled with empty calories, these items simply ooze saturated fat. They also load these things up with preservatives to prolong shelf life in the frozen foods section of supermarkets. There are some that are better than others, but there is no reason you should ever be hard up enough, or so pressed for time, that you must opt for this crap over a decent meal.

Alternatives: In the time it takes to heat up the oven, or read the microwave directions and wait for the timer to go off, you could open a can of sockeye salmon and plunk the contents down in the middle of a bed of organic, baby greens, and have it with a slice of rye or pumpernickel bread, washed down with organic green tea. Okay, it's not pizza, but you are looking to get rid of your pizza- and beer-gut anyway.

Processed white bread: Any product which contains enriched white flour as its primary ingredient is definitely off your list of desirable foods from now on. Enriched only means all the goodness has been taken out of the natural wheat during the processing and bleaching stage, and that vitamins and other nutrients had to be added artificially afterward in order to put some of the goodness back. There is almost no fibre content, and it is filled with preservatives to keep it fresh on the grocer's shelves for a week or longer. In fact, sometimes it gets mouldy and it's still soft when you squeeze it. What does this tell you about what's in it?

Alternatives: Whole grain bread and rolls made with organically grown, sprouted grains, if possible. If not, choose either rye bread - the darker, the better - or pumpernickel, all of which have plenty of fibre. The latter two also help increase the body's metabolic rate, while the fibre in all of these can help the body eliminate toxins and bad cholesterol from the arteries.

Instant rice: Like its close cousin, processed white bread, instant rice, or instant anything, means it has been heat-processed, then freeze-dried, so that it can be reconstituted quickly with the application of boiling water. There is next to no nutritional benefit eating this stuff, but there are plenty of detrimental effects on your body. Pure starch, no fibre, and no vitamins, unless they've been added after the fact. White rice, and especially instant white rice, also has a very high glycemic index.

Alternatives: Organically grown long-grain or short-grain brown rice; organically grown brown Basmati rice; and a number of nutritionally sound, delicious rices which can easily be purchased at your health food store or from any bulk food store. Even some supermarkets are carrying these alternatives now, so take a look around. It takes about a half hour to cook any rice, and that's not much longer than it takes to get the instant variety prepared anyway.

Doughnuts: How many reasons do you need to stay away from this kind of poison? Enriched white flour, rancid fat, sugar coming out the ying-yang . . . filled with empty calories, trans-fatty acids, simple carbohydrates, and virtually no nutritional benefit. This is the kind of eating habit that puts inches around your middle and creates serious health problems. Heard enough, or should I get more graphic?

Alternatives: Low-fat, sugar-free organic oat bran or wheat bran muffins, but nothing else. Most of the time the muffins found in these doughnut chain stores are as unhealthy and fattening as the doughnuts. Stay away from these places and find a good vegetarian restaurant that sells good healthy muffins, as well.

Chinese food: Do you really think the people who live in China eat this kind of food? Hardly. They've concocted most of these recipes to suit North American tastes for sugar, fat and white flour. Most entrees feature breaded, deep-fried foods which have loads of fat and are brimming with trans-fatty acids just waiting to do a number on your arterial system and your internal organs. To add injury to insult, they usually load everything up with monosodium glutamate (MSG) - a highly carcinogenic chemical that supposedly brings out the taste and leaves vegetables looking colourful long after they've had the goodness boiled, steamed, and fried out of them. Even the fried rice has too much fat and too many empty calories, and once they start piling on the sweet and sour sauces, you might as well be eating doughnuts. Stay away from egg rolls and spring rolls, too, because they are nothing more than deep-fried grease traps.

Alternatives: Vietnamese restaurants generally stay away from deep-fried food, serving sauté chicken and beef instead, with hot and spicy dipping sauces. They usually serve steamed rice, and their vegetables are stir-fried to a nice, crunchy texture. Generally they don't use MSG, but ask them not to, just in case. Choose the Vietnamese salad rolls, which feature fresh salad and veggies and sometimes shrimp, rolled inside rice-paper skins.

Potato chips: Commercial potato chips, cheese corn, and a variety of similar products are some of the major contributors to bad health and abuse of the medical system in North America today. Almost completely devoid of any nutritional content, they contain high levels of trans-fatty acids, high-cholesterol saturated fats and high levels of sodium. Whatever goodness was originally in these vegetables - potatoes and corn - is completely lost in the process of turning them into snack foods. Kids all over North America are ruining the foundation of their health with this crap, and if you are a middle-aged man eating these things.... well, if someone told you to jump off a building, would you do that, too, simply because it was easy or because it tasted good?

Alternatives: Carrot, celery and zucchini sticks make excellent snack foods, and they are every bit as crunchy as potato chips. If you must, try organically grown, stone-ground tortilla chips that are baked, not fried, and dip them into organic refried beans. There is enough nutritional goodness, fibre, vitamins and minerals in meals of tortilla chips and beans to be a complete meal, if you only add an organic salad on the side.

Canned foods: With a few notable exceptions, almost anything that comes in a can is not worth opening. Vegetables have had the goodness cooked out of them at the ultra-high temperatures used in the canning process. Fruits are in the same category, but have had high-sugar syrup added, along with artificial fruit flavouring to make up for the shortfall that occurs during processing. And don't get me started on those canned pasta products, nor the stews, soups, and other quick meal ideas. To make matters worse, canners also use heavy doses of MSG to keep colour in fruits and veggies.

Alternatives: You can find fruits packed in their own juice, and they do put organic fruit and vegetables in cans these days as well; these are a reasonable alternative, as long as you aren't using them as your dietary staples. Some exceptions to the can rule is canned fish like salmon, sardines, and tuna (packed in water, not highly salted vegetable broth).

Fast food franchises: The quickest way to become an invalid in your senior years - if you live that long - is to buy into the advertising campaigns that have made these franchises wealthy at the expense of North Americans' health. There are no acceptable hamburgers, cheeseburgers, fish burgers, chicken burgers, french fries, onion rings or any of the other patented poisons these places dispense on a continual basis. Some even have breaded, deep-fried process cheese bits. Any of the marquee burgers advertised by the major franchises contain a day's supply of saturated fat, not to mention enough nitrites, trans-fatty acids and toxic chemicals to kill your will to live. If you can't learn to say "no thank you," to this kind of stuff, you may as well start prepaying your funeral arrangements now. If you have been eating this stuff, it's unlikely you can see your own feet when you look towards the floor.

Alternatives: There are none. Truthfully, if we, as middle-aged men in North America, can't find enough will power to stop eating this so-called "food," then what hope is there that the future generations will be in better shape? We're teaching them the eating habits they need to be in even worse condition, worse shape. Can we leave this earth shouldering this kind of guilt?

Okay, if you must eat fast food, and it's highly recommended that you never, ever do, then try the Mexican alternatives, which feature veggie burritos (the "tastiest" item on these menus). Some places feature baked potatoes, which are fine as long as you don't load them up with sour cream, butter (or margarine) and bacon bits. Some offer a salad bar, though you have to ignore the high-fat dressings. Nothing else will do.

Chapter 3
Free Radicals and Anti-Oxidants

The presence of uncontrolled free radicals in the body is the direct cause of many health problems that are on the increase these days. Free radicals are "loose cannon" molecules that are constantly making us sick, causing us to age prematurely, and which will eventually contribute heavily to our demise.

A free radical is an atom or molecule with an unpaired electron. Unless you understand organic chemistry, which I don't, a deeper explanation isn't necessary. All you really need to know is that this condition is a hazardous, unstable, and unnatural state. This odd, unpaired electron in the free radical causes it to collide with other molecules and steal an electron from them. When this happens, it changes the structure of these other molecules and causes them to also become free radicals. This, in turn, creates a self-perpetuating chain reaction, in which the structure of millions of molecules is altered. Bottom line, it's a bad situation.

Everything from age spots, to wrinkles, to Alzheimer's disease can be traced to free radical damage in our bodies. Free oxygen radicals, the main type formed in living organisms, have also been implicated in disorders such as heart disease, cataracts, and rheumatoid arthritis. They also contribute greatly to the physiological processes associated with growing old, such as wrinkling of the skin, the decline of kidney function, and increased susceptibility to autoimmune diseases.

Free radicals occur naturally as by-products of biochemical reactions that occur in normal metabolic functions. They also enter our bodies through the food we eat, in our water supplies, drugs and medicines we ingest, and in the air we breath. The environment also contributes immensely to the spread of free radicals, as do processes like drugs, radiation, pesticides, air pollutants, solvents, fried foods, alcohol, tobacco smoke and many other things we are all exposed to on a regular basis.

Cigarette smoking is a major producer of oxidants, both for those who smoke and for those exposed to the second-hand smoke in the environment.

As a defence against free radicals, our bodies produce something called anti-oxidants or "free radical scavengers." These anti-oxidants neutralize free radicals by sacrificing an electron to the free radical, which then becomes paired with the formerly unpaired electron, thereby stabilizing the free radical - sort of like finding dance partners for all the singles. Nevertheless, it is this balance between free radicals and antioxidants that has guaranteed our survival for thousands of years.

Although the body does produce its own anti-oxidants, it also makes use of anti-oxidant nutrients and phytochemicals we ingest, most especially in vitamins E, C and beta-carotene, as well as the minerals selenium and zinc.

Studies have shown that vigorous exercise increases the production of free radicals because as athletes, we tend to use more oxygen, since exercise increases our rate of breathing. Therefore, athletes need to ensure that their diets include plenty of antioxidant-producing fruits and vegetables as well as daily supplements. As a part of your healthy, active lifestyle, increase your intake of fruit, vegetables and vitamin supplements. To make matters simpler, choose fruits and vegetables with plenty of colour - preferably ones which have been organically grown since pesticides, herbicides, chemical fertilizers and the like tend to create even more free radicals; the deeper the colour, the more powerful the antioxidants.

Here's a breakdown of the most powerful antioxidants and where to find them on a daily basis. For those who are too nutritionally challenged to find the antioxidants in their naturally occurring state, most of these compounds can be found in pill and capsule form at your neighbourhood natural food store:

Lycopene: is the red pigment found in tomatoes and berries and has proven to be more a more potent antioxidant than vitamin E and beta carotene.

Beta Carotene: is found in carrots, sweet potatoes, pumpkin, broccoli, cantaloupe and mangos.

Vitamin C: is found in red and green bell peppers, broccoli, cauliflower, strawberries, spinach, potatoes, and citrus fruits.

Vitamin E: is found in almonds, soybeans, and raw sunflower seeds.

Selenium: is found in white tuna (choose the kind that's packed in water, not oil or vegetable broth), sunflower seeds, and whole grains.

Some other powerful antioxidants you can take as supplements on a daily basis include pycnogenol, which is derived from the bark of European pine trees; grape seed extract; and green tea - either Japanese or Chinese, preferably organically grown.

Chlorophyll: also acts as an antioxidant, and dark green vegetables, including wheat grass and barley grass, contain phytochemicals that may offer additional antioxidant protection.

The daily consumption of dark green leafy vegetables is strongly recommended, since it's these foods which provide the body with a generous supply of folic acid, vitamin K, magnesium, carotenoids, iron, trace minerals. and chlorophyll.

The fibre, vitamin K, and chlorophyll content found in green vegetables also work together to promote a favourable balance of friendly bacteria, which benefits intestinal health. And digestive health is considered the cornerstone of optimal nutrition.

Dietary anti-oxidants help:

- maximize life span

- prevent cell damage

- slow the aging process

- speed healing of wounds

- prevent arthritis

- protect against heart disease

- prevent cancer

- eliminate allergies

- prevent mental deterioration

Acidity and Alkalinity

The act of balancing the PH level in our bodily fluids is achieved by eating the proper balance of acid and alkaline foods. PH stands for potential of hydrogen and is a scale used to measure the relative acidity or alkalinity of substances.

PH levels are measured on a scale ranging from 0 through 14, with zero being completely acidic and 14 being completely alkaline. The average PH level in our bodies is somewhere in the 7.0 range, although this is an average of extremes, fluctuating between highly acidic gastric fluids of the stomach, which can tip the PH scales at anywhere from 1.0 to 3.5 - so they can break up and digest the foods we eat, and the arterial blood, which may range from 7.35 to 7.45. With 7 being neutral, numbers higher than that indicate an increase in alkalinity, while numbers below 7 indicate an increase in acidity.

Although the arterial blood range may seem very narrow, bear in mind that these numbers, much like those associated with the Richter scale for measuring earthquakes, increase exponentially. A PH level of 7 is 10 times greater than a level of 6 and 8 is 100 times greater than 6 and so on.

The purpose of these numbers is only to illustrate how small changes in PH levels within our bodily fluids can have a dramatic result on our overall wellness. If the PH of arterial blood slips below 7.3, we slip into convulsions, and death is imminent.

If we are consuming a well-balanced, nutritionally complete diet each and every day, drinking enough pure water so our bodies can buffer the acidity to keep us in proper balance, then we can easily maintain the right PH level. However, if we are typical North Americans, we are consuming too many acidifying foods, which throws the body out of balance. An overabundance of these foods creates an acidic environment in which our health suffers quickly.

When we become too acidic, there are a great number of chemical and physiological changes that occur which are detrimental to our health. The worst damage comes from increased free radical oxidation, which occurs with greater ease, while antioxidant activity becomes impaired. The result of this process is simply that we age much faster.

Meanwhile, our athletic performance decreases as the muscles produce more ammonia. along with more lactic and pyruvic acids. These acids decrease muscle contraction and expansion, and less oxygen is available to the cells. This occurs naturally when we exercise our muscles vigorously, producing these acids, which decrease the ability of the muscles to function. Hence we get to a point of exhaustion when we either can't run any longer, or can't perform another repetition in the gymnasium.

The permeability of cell walls is also lessened when our bodies become acidic, and this inhibits absorption of vitamins and minerals. Connective tissue also becomes weakened, which results in loss of tone and texture to the skin and hair.

This is also a time when colds, infections and a host of other maladies become common, since there is a toxic buildup and cells are biologically stressed.

Ideally, in order to maintain a neutral PH within our bodies, we must try and consume more foods that are alkalizing over foods that are acidifying, in a ratio of about three to one. This means about 75 per cent of our daily nutritional intake should be alkalizing foods.

In general, the North American diet is heavily balanced in the other direction, thanks to the abundance of modified, overprocessed, fast foods, and foods designed with flavour and convenience as the key factors, rather than nutritional content. Because of this trend, degenerative diseases such as cancers, osteoporosis, arthritis and immune dysfunction, to name a few, are rampant. It is also clear why so many North Americans are in such bad shape and such poor condition.

The acidifying foods include all oils, even the organically grown, cold-pressed varieties such as hemp seed, flax seed, sunflower, sesame, safflower, olive, and the essential blends like Udo's Choice and Essential Balance. Butter, margarine, lard, shortening and even vegetable oil sprays, too.

All grains are acidifying, and that goes especially for rice cakes and wheat cakes. So, too, are all dairy products, with the exception of fat-free, plain yoghurt. This includes cheeses of all varieties, with the exception of fat-free cottage cheese.

With the exception of almonds and chestnuts, all nuts and nut butters are also on the acidifying side of the chart, as is all animal-based protein, with the exception of lean, skinless chicken breasts.

All sweets, sugars, and sugar-sweetened foods are acidifying as well. This includes molasses and honey, aspartame, saccharin and maple syrup; also included are all alcoholic beverages, including all wines. Drugs, chemicals, both prescription and otherwise, are on this list as well, and so are all beans and legumes. Some of the others include all distilled varieties of vinegar.

The list is long, but fortunately the list of alkalizing foods is even longer. All vegetables are part of the alkalizing group as are all fruits, with the exception of cranberries. Cranberries do not stimulate the pancreas like other fruits do, but carry an antibiotic that works only in an acidic environment.

From the protein group, the alkalizing ones include free-range eggs, skinless chicken breasts, and whey protein powder. Plain, non-fat yogurt is also a good source of protein, as is tofu. Sunflower seeds, pumpkin seeds, flax seeds and squash seeds are all alkalizing, as are all sprouted seeds and nuts. The only grain which makes this list, is millet, and the only nut on the list is the almond.

Apple cider vinegar is, of course, alkalizing, while so too are most spices and seasonings, as well as herbs, lecithin granules, bee pollen and dairy-free probiotic cultures.

Alkalizing beverages include all fresh fruit and vegetable juices (not pre-packaged, fruit-flavoured ones, though), organic, unpasteurized milk and purified or distilled water. Herbal teas, including green tea, are also on the alkalizing side of the chart, but the only sweetener on this side is one called stevia. Stevia is a potent South American herbal sweetener also grown in the Orient. Just a pinch of stevia - also known as honeyleaf - is as sweet as a heaping tablespoon of other sweeteners, and there are almost no calories. It is also a low-glycemic food and does not raise insulin levels.

Black coffee, not decaffeinated, is also alkalizing, which is somewhat of a surprise. However, it becomes acidic once you sweeten it with anything other than stevia and, again, if you put cream, milk, or a petroleum whitener in it. It should also be consumed with meals, because if you drink it on an empty stomach, it has an acidifying effect.

If you suspect your body is still acidic even after you have changed your diet to this three-to-one ratio of alkalizing foods, you may want to supplement with magnesium and potassium, both of which will raise the PH level.

It will take a period of time - perhaps as much as four to six weeks, or as few as two or three - before you have built up your alkaline reserves and your body fluids gain their proper acid-alkaline balance, which is known as homeostasis. Once this has occurred, your sleep patterns should get back to normal range, and you'll have a greater supply of natural energy. You should also suffer far less from the colds, headaches, infections and flu's that plague ordinary North Americans.

All of this will benefit you greatly in the gym as well, and will make the task of rebuilding your body easier.

Smoking and Alcohol Consumption

This may sound like a no-brainer, but if you are a smoker, quit. Right now. No amount of advice in this book or any other is going to be able to compensate for the 4,000+ deadly chemicals and toxins you are sucking into your body up to 50 or 60 times daily. If you haven't got at least as much personal discipline as it takes to give up smoking, there's no point in going any further.

If you are of the belief that smoking is not going to affect you, or somehow hasn't affected you up to this point, think again. Almost half the patient load in hospitals across North America is as a result of smoking - either directly or indirectly. Every time you inhale cigarette smoke, you are impairing the ability of every organ in your body to function properly. What's more, you're destroying the largest organ in the human body - the skin. Smoking will add years to your appearance and, in case you haven't caught the drift here, that's the exact opposite of what we're trying to accomplish.

Lung cancer and a large percentage of colon cancer, as well as a significant number of other cancers, can be attributed to cigarette smoking. Once you quit, your chance of getting cancer will slowly abate until, after a certain period - as much as 10-to-15 years in some cases- the ex-smoker's risk is comparable to people who have never smoked.

In the face of overwhelming evidence pointing out the risks attributed to smoking, it's a wonder so many still choose to indulge. Cigars and pipes can be equally as bad, perhaps worse, since the amount of nicotine and other toxins contained in a single cigar is equivalent to as much as a half a pack of cigarettes or more. Ditto for pipe smoking.

Worse still is the habit of chewing tobacco and/or putting snuff between your lip and gums. While this may never result in lung cancer, it will certainly make you a candidate for all manner of skin, gum, tongue, and glandular cancers in the region of your mouth and throat.

The same can be said for the consumption of alcohol. Besides the obvious detriment to your health that comes with drinking - liver and kidney problems, deterioration of brain cells and so on - alcohol also acts as an inhibitor for a great many trace elements, vitamins and enzymes. Drinking even a moderate amount each day can put your entire body out of equilibrium.

There is one exception, and that is the consumption of red wine, which can actually be beneficial to your health, provided it is consumed in moderation.

Few people have likely heard of a phenomenon known as "the French paradox," whereby the French have a lower rate of cardiovascular disease, in spite of a diet that is typically high in fat. It is actually the flavenoids in red wine that are to be thanked for saving the French from themselves.

Unfortunately, it isn't the alcohol that is the catalyst, so there is no redeeming value to drinking. The same flavenoids are also present in ordinary grape juice. These potent antioxidants protect against the oxidation of LDL cholesterol and they can also prevent platelet aggregation, which lowers the risk of dangerous blood clots.

As if you needed yet another reason to give up alcohol, think about the acidifying effects it is having on your body.

Chapter 4
Detoxification

After years of poor eating habits - particularly the ingestion of too much red meat and too many processed foods containing additives - there will be an accumulation of debris and undigested food in your bowels. If you haven't paid attention to the quality of water you've been drinking, there is likely a buildup of heavy metals in your muscle tissue, too. This is basically what's known as toxicity and it's important to try and rid your body of as much of this deadly matter as possible in order to rebuild from the inside out.

Therefore, it's important to go through a brief or even a lengthy period of detoxification if you hope to give yourself a fighting chance for the future.

It's somewhat like organic gardening, in that the grower must first ensure the ground is certified organic. To do this, he embarks on a three-to-five-year plan of soil detoxification, during which no pesticides, herbicides, fungicides, or chemical fertilizers are added to the soil. In the meantime, they add organic compost and rich, decaying vegetable matter to the ground, to replenish the minerals lost to years of growing crops with inorganic processes.

What you want to do is to make your ground as clean, organic and fertile as possible so that all your bodily functions can return to normal including your digestive tract, circulatory and immune systems. At the same time, ridding yourself of this toxic debris will aid in mental acuity, and mental wellness in general.

Depending on how deep and how cleansed you want to be, this process can be long and complicated - such as chelation therapy, for example - or it can take place within your home, on your own terms, using a form of chelation and dieting.

Chelation is a process whereby a formula containing a protein-like molecule is added to the body intravenously. This formula draws out the heavy metals from within the muscle fibres because the molecule binds to metal ions, making them soluble in blood. These metals - cadmium, calcium, copper, mercury and lead - are then moved to the kidneys where they can be excreted. This process sometimes takes weeks or even months of continuous applications and can be very costly. Nevertheless, it can help rid the body of deadly toxins and heavy metals at a molecular level.

Most patients experience minimal or no side affects during the process of chelation and there are a host of long-term benefits when it has been completed such as better skin colour, more rapid wound healing, improved memory, increased energy, improved kidney function, improved vision and a host of others.

On the other hand, there are simpler ways to help rid the body of toxins. One of these is to simply go on a brief fruit and vegetable juice fast, followed up with a day or two of eating organic, raw foods containing plenty of fibre.

One method goes something like this: upon rising, on an empty stomach, drink an eight-to-10-ounce glass of either purified or distilled water to which a teaspoonful of sodium sulphate has been added. Sodium sulphate, or Glauber salts, as they were once known, are still available through a pharmacy or at your local health food store.

This saline solution will not only empty your bowels in short order, but in the process will draw toxic matter, heavy metals and body waste into the bowels from all parts of the body. The elimination process will be messy and putrid, but will do wonders for your entire system.

When this is done, it should be followed up by drinking several litres of fresh citrus fruit juice - a combination of grapefruit, orange and lemon. These fruits should be organically grown if at all possible. Don't drink this juice all in one sitting, but take an eight-ounce glassful every half hour or so beginning a half hour after taking the saline solution. Try not to eat anything for the entire day, but drink plenty of purified or distilled water instead to help in the process of elimination. If you can last the entire day, by the following day you'll feel like a new man... essentially because you will be!

Also that following day, try to eat nothing but raw fruits and vegetables - again, preferably organic - and eat only organic salad with a dressing of essential oil and apple cider vinegar with a bit of Spike added for taste. You can also drink vegetable juices that you can either purchase from a vendor, or make yourself at home using a juicer.

Juices from fruits and vegetable contain all the enzymes, nutrients, minerals and amino acids necessary to sustain life. These are easily digested in a matter of minutes as opposed to eating cooked food, which can remain in the digestive tract for many hours before being broken down and processed into the necessary nutrients. Fruit and vegetable juices also contain organic water, which can be absorbed immediately into the cells.

A valuable compound is activated charcoal - either in powder or capsule form, with the latter being by far the easiest to ingest. Charcoal is a supreme cleanser of the body because it is very porous and so has a large surface area to adsorb (attract and hold) toxins from within the body. Charcoal will adsorb chemicals, drugs, gases, body wastes and foreign proteins.

Activated charcoal is made by the controlled burning of the source material, then subjected to a stream of air at high temperatures which causes a network of internal pores that greatly increase its surface area and adsorptive capabilities. Charcoal capsules or tablets are available in most pharmacies and all health food stores and cost very little.

Taking activated charcoal capsules will also cure heartburn, indigestion and gas problems in the intestinal tract very quickly and very efficiently. They will also alleviate flatulence, since they can absorb 80 times their weight in gas - hence their use in gas masks.

Charcoal adsorbs a large number of toxins extremely well, including radioactive substances, pesticides, narcotics, iodine, chlordane, alcohol, morphine and acetaminophen.

If you are eating highly cleansing food or juices for a period of time, one of the side affects is diarrhea. This may make you feel uncomfortable for a day or so, but it is extremely valuable as a method of ridding the body and the bowels of the putrid waste matter that has been flushed out of your system. It's not something to be alarmed about, unless it continues for more than

68

48 hours, at which time you may want to consult a physician. However, a few charcoal capsules will almost always cure any case of diarrhea.

A simple detoxification using fruit and vegetable juice should never result in prolonged diarrhea, so don't worry.

Ironically, you will likely also experience another side affect of juice fasting and cleansing - a burst of energy. In spite of the fact that you won't be eating the usual foods, your energy level should be elevated, and you'll feel better than you ever did previously. And it's just the start!

Health food stores also specialize in colon and intestinal cleansing formulas that are usually three-to-five-day plans, sometimes as much as 10 days or even two weeks. They also do a very effective job of eliminating putrid waste matter from the body. They come with easy-to-follow directions, and I know of a good number of people who have successfully completed these cleanses, and sing their praises.

Removing heavy metals is important, but so is the removal of toxic trace minerals, because these generally tend to replace the good trace minerals in our bodies, unless they are flushed out.

The most toxic of these include aluminum, arsenic, cadmium, lead and mercury.

In large doses, aluminum can cause bone abnormalities, muscle weakness, loss of balance and co-ordination, memory loss and depression. Because it interferes with the absorption of important minerals such as selenium, magnesium and calcium, it can bring on diseases, which are caused by a lack of these minerals.

Aluminum is a byproduct of industry, passed through smokestacks, dumped into rivers and waste sites, and brought down to earth in the form of acid rain. It also enters water through municipal treatment plants, because aluminum sulfate (alum) is used to clarify the water. Adding fluoride to drinking water makes the aluminum even more toxic, because it makes it more difficult to excrete.

Aluminum is also commonly used as an emulsifier, to prevent clumping in processed foods such as flours, baking powder, processed fruits and vegetables, and table salt. There are dozens of variations on aluminum additives, but some of the more common ones you'll find on food labels are alum, aluminum potassium sulfate, sodium aluminum phosphate, sodium silicon aluminate, aluminum calcium silicate, potassium alum, aluminum stearate, and aluminum hydroxide which is common in drugstore antiperspirants and deodorants.

Excess arsenic can cause high blood pressure, skin abnormalities such as odd pigmentation, lesions and psoriasis, diarrhea, indigestion, cancer and poor circulation. This is also some evidence that it can be a factor in causing diabetes.

Cadmium is not only toxic on its own, but displaces zinc, one of our most important trace minerals. It also blocks the absorption of iron, and overexposure to cadmium also causes lung, kidney and liver disease, high blood pressure, and may play a role in Alzheimer's disease.

The effects of lead poisoning are subtle, and lead to deterioration of the brain. Sufficient supplements of calcium and magnesium can prevent lead poisoning, since an absence of these minerals causes the body to take up lead instead. A source of lead poisoning is old plumbing, which has lead soldering and so poisons the tap water.

Symptoms of lead poisoning can include confusion, headaches, constipation, fatigue, weight loss, high blood pressure, kidney disease, degenerative brain diseases and digestive problems. In fact, it's a lot like waking up with a hangover.

Overexposure to lead is linked with cancer, because it interferes with the production of glutathione, the body's first level of antioxidant defence.

Mercury is one of the most toxic of the heavy metals, as it inhibits the body's use of the B vitamin folic acid. It also alters protein structures, which are involved in every aspect of bodily function.

Mercury is another common by-product of industrial wastes, and is also a common waste product in hospitals. It is often dumped into the waterways or oceans, and can there be ingested by fish.

Larger fish, such as tuna and swordfish, which live near the coastal areas, often have very high levels of mercury in their flesh.

Symptoms of mercury poisoning include central nervous system damage, such as is seen in multiple sclerosis and Alzheimer's disease. Other symptoms include insomnia, anorexia, chronic fatigue, depression, headaches, diarrhea, irregular heartbeat, hair loss, irritability, kidney damage, loss of sex drive and muscle weakness. Mercury also suppresses the immune system.

Antacids

Stomach problems are fairly common among North American men these days. This is especially so if they are eating on the run, eating out a lot at fast food establishments, or are simply ingesting a lot of overprocessed foods with a high-acid content. As a result, antacid tablets have become one of the most popular non-prescription medicinal aids in history. People eat millions of these little tablets daily, hoping to ease their upset stomachs or quell bouts of heartburn and/or acid indigestion. Antacids weaken or neutralize stomach acid for a brief period, relieving these symptoms, but they often reappear or rebound as the stomach tries to make up for the stomach acid it doesn't have by working overtime.

These tablets are now popularly advertised as a good source of calcium. In truth, they can actually deplete the body of calcium, since the aluminum and magnesium in the antacids tends to bind with phosphate, which can result in calcium depletion.

Antacids usually deliver large doses of aluminum hydroxides, which are among the worst culprits for blocking mineral absorption. If taken with citrus fruits or citrus drinks, the amount of aluminum that is absorbed is increased.

If you need an antacid, and you likely won't have to worry about this once you are eating a properly balanced diet and more wholesome foods, try using activated charcoal capsules. Better still, take a tablespoon or two of apple cider vinegar in a little warm water. This works quickly and more effectively than any antacid tablet on the market, and the only side affects are the beneficial ones you get when you take this wonderful compound.

Rebuilding

After detoxification, a balanced, nutritious diet, plenty of purified water, strenuous exercise such as body building and taking daily vitamin supplements will make a big difference in your body's ability to clear out any overload of toxic minerals.

After a cleanse like this, it's also a good idea to immediately begin a program of probiotics to introduce new "friendly" bacteria to the gut and intestinal tract. Friendly bacteria such as acidophilus and bifidus, and a number of others, aid in the digestion of food and absorption of enzymes. At some time, almost everyone has been on antibiotics. When used properly and sparingly, they can be a powerful weapon against infection. Unfortunately, antibiotics indiscriminately kill all forms of bacteria in the human body, including the friendly bacteria of the digestive tract. For example, the B-complex vitamin biotin is produced by just such friendly bacteria in the gut.

Some antibiotics can also inhibit the absorption of calcium, iron, and potassium, as well as vitamin B-12, while others, such as those known as quinlones, will block the absorption of calcium, iron, and zinc.

Probiotics can be purchased at health food stores, while foods that contain living bacteria cultures - such as organic yoghurt, kefir and sour milk - are also beneficial in replacing the friendly bacteria necessary for proper digestion and mineral absorption.

It would also be a good time to introduce enzymes and herbs that will aid in rebuilding the immune system, such as Echinacea, zinc and garlic.

Chapter 5
Out of the jungle and into the gym

Some men reach mid life and are still working at a job that requires they be physically active. However, there aren't a lot of these guys about. If you're like most middle-aged men, you spend a great deal of your life sitting - at a desk, in a car, in a plane, watching television and so on. Even those who begin their working careers in a position of manual labour have likely worked their way up the ladder of success to attain a senior position - one which likely requires less physical exertion than it does mental anxiety.

Sitting for long periods is counterproductive to good health. (duh!) Your joints and lower back stiffen, your circulation becomes impaired, and your metabolism slows considerably. Prolonged inactivity eventually causes the immune system to deteriorate, and it robs the body of its vital capacity. It also reduces motivation.

To get things back on track requires exercise - not just casual, physical activity, but the kind of pulse-quickening endeavour that makes you break sweat while elevating your heart rate.

Exercise, particularly the weight-lifting variety, combined with optimum diet and the use of dietary supplements will help you successfully develop an overall better fat-muscle ratio body composition.

Walking or even a round of golf may be therapeutic, but it won't prevent the atrophy of muscle that is observed in men and women as they age - something known as sarcopenia. Walking isn't strenuous enough to trigger the release of growth hormones or to elevate testosterone levels - two powerful hormones that decline with age, but which are necessary to prevent muscles from atrophying. Only strenuous physical activity elevates these important hormonal levels.

There is now a synthetic testosterone available through prescription from your family doctor, and a lot of men have apparently found it helps them regain some of their lost youth. On the other hand, there are dangerous side affects, including the potential for liver disease and cancer of liver that are greatly elevated by the use of these synthetic hormones.

Then too, there are the emotional side effects, which, according to some users, are equivalent to premenstrual syndrome in women. We don't even want to go there!

Alternatively, there are certain herbal supplements available that can help your body trigger the production of testosterone, and these are safer and more easily acquired. If you need to get your testosterone kick-started, a product called "Testostergain," marketed by a company called ProNutrient Supplements, is available in tablet form. There are likely a number of similar products under different brand names, marketed by a variety of nutritional supplement companies, so check around and ask questions at your local gym or health food store. Users take one tablet three times a day during a 21-day "cycle," and then take a week off before going through two more "cycles."

The results range from hardly noticeable to fairly dramatic, especially where shedding fat and gaining lean muscle are concerned. The results are directly linked to the amount of testosterone that is lacking in your body, so those who produce the least would benefit the most from these products, while those who are still producing considerable quantities of their own would not benefit nearly so much, and the results would be less dramatic.

On the other hand, these supplements are not a "quick fix," and if you are looking for ways to cut corners in your quest for fitness and well being, don't bother with these until such time as you've toned up and slimmed down, and have a well-established fitness routine working for you. Shortcuts are for kids who go to gyms to get huge bodies in as brief a period of time as possible.

Some of these so-called bodybuilders will inject themselves with anabolic steroids, in an effort to get the kind of gains which ordinarily would take months or even longer to accomplish.

Steroids function in a manner similar to testosterone, the male hormone chiefly responsible for muscle growth. There is a terrible price they will pay for their careless desire to look muscular at any cost. The long-term side effects of anabolic steroid use can be devastating, and will last much longer than the muscle they hope to gain along the way. Liver damage and a decrease in the size of their testicles, thereby interfering with their reproductive system, are some of the common long-term affects. Prolonged use can also result in hair loss, and reportedly produces a rapid lowering of HDL cholesterol - the type that is necessary for proper body function.

However, we are looking to improve your lifestyle and your way of life, not to add to what may be an already lengthy list of complications brought on by years of bad living and neglect. Remember, if it isn't a solution, it's just another problem.

A long, slow program of muscle building produces high quality tissue that will look better and perform more efficiently. The longer the process, the more the tendons and sinews have a chance to adjust to the additional muscle. Besides, steroid users end up with outrageous muscle bulk, often having shoulders in different time zones. You don't want to be a muscle freak. A well-toned, muscular physique is far more attractive, and draws more attention, than the spectacle of someone who has blown themselves out of proportion using pharmaceutical enhancements.

If you want to remain lean for life, you have to find and follow a program that keeps up your basal metabolic rate (BMR). This is the minimum amount of energy your body expends to maintain vital processes like respiration, circulation and digestion. Sitting will sabotage your fat-burning potential, and your thyroid gland adapts to this sedentary lifestyle by adjusting your internal thermostat, which then turns you into a fat-storing machine. Inactivity accelerates loss of lean mass and cardiac function. As they say, "you lose what you do not use."

Without an exercise program, after age 20 you start to lose vibrant, fat-burning muscle while strength, stamina and bone density decrease. To worsen matters, your blood pressure, cholesterol and triglycerides increase during this process. You start to get heavier as you get older, while at the same time you begin experiencing fatigue, chronic pain, and stress.

Besides the aesthetic value, there are other, more important reasons for wanting to build muscle mass. It is a fact that reduced muscle mass and strength leads to a slower metabolism, an increase in body fat, less aerobic capacity, and loss of bone tissue density.

Exercise can increase your muscle mass, benefiting your body in many ways. The ratio of muscle to fat in our bodies helps to determine our metabolic rate, our aerobic capacity, and the ratio of beneficial HDL-cholesterol levels. Studies show that we can lose an average of 30 per cent of muscle mass from age 20 through age 70. However, biopsies performed on the muscles of older men, who did lifelong strength training, looked the same as those of 25-year olds. The same biopsies performed on sedentary men, as well as those who only participated in aerobic-style training, showed typical age-related changes. The bottom line is that you can build some strength in certain parts of your body through aerobic training - legs in running or cycling, arms, shoulders, back and legs in cross-country skiing - but you need a muscle-strengthening program to ensure continued strength as you drift into the later stages of life.

Therefore, the smart thing to do is to build muscle mass, and the only way to do this is through a system of weight-bearing exercises and proper eating habits. So, if you've never seen the inside of a gym, now is a perfect time to get started.

If you absolutely refuse to join a gym, don't have one handy or for some other reason simply can't be bothered, there are other ways of working out - the home gym, for instance - and we'll cover those areas a little later on.

Although it really doesn't matter what kind of gymnasium you join, the smartest thing you could do for yourself, especially if you're not accustomed to going to the gym, is to make certain it is close to either your home or your place of employment. The reason for this is that if it is close at hand, you will be more likely to use it more often than if it is across town or in some out-of-the way place. You'd be surprised at how often people take out memberships in a gym, only to quit going after just a few sessions because it's too difficult to get to or because it is too out of the way to be convenient. It's been said many times before that the best gym is one that you'll use.

The best idea is one known as the 15-minute formula. If the gym is more than 15 minutes by car or by foot, from either your home or your office, then find something closer.

Getting started

There are a few important points to remember just before getting started on a fitness/workout routine, especially if you have never previously worked out or have led a very sedentary life up to this point.

First, if you are run down, overweight and already have a history of heart and/or respiratory problems, you might want to consider hiring a personal trainer for the first week or two. This will help you to get a good program in place and to get some valuable pointers about the correct procedure for lifting free weights and some instruction on the use of those fancy and sometimes complicated pieces of machinery you'll find in the gyms.

A lot of fitness magazines and books will encourage you to see your family doctor before embarking on a new fitness program. Why bother? What's he going to tell you - that you can't become physically fit, or that he doesn't recommend you try and get in shape? If you do see a doctor, and he says he doesn't recommend you go to a gym, find another doctor. Better still, invite him to come along. It'll probably do him a world of good as well.

Besides, if you or your doctor think you might expire on a treadmill during your first visit, what's to prevent you from dying while walking from the parking lot to the office?

And, don't ever begin a workout without first going through a proper warm-up. This means at least eight-to-10 minutes on either a stationary bike, a stairstepper, a treadmill or some other cardio device. Better yet, a brisk walk for 10 or 15 minutes to the gym (carrying your gym strip, of course) will do nicely, as will either riding your bike or inline skating to the gym.

This warm-up period will get the blood flowing in your veins, get your heart rate up a bit and will warm up every muscle in your body properly before you begin lifting free weights or using the machinery.

Going at it cold - without a proper warm-up period - will result in possible muscle and/or tendon injury and will leave you with a lot more pain and stiffness the following day.

Since you will be combining an aerobic workout with your weight resistance training, wait until after you have completed your resistance weight training before moving on to your cardio work. Spend at least 20-30 minutes doing a cardio workout; whether it is on a road bike, stationary bike, inline skates, or whatever is your personal choice. Combine a cardio workout either with your weight training or do it separately on alternate days. Do cardio at least three times a week, in addition to your weight training. The combination of weights and aerobic workout works faster than anything else to build muscle and burn fat.

The Workout

When you're working out, each time you lift a weight it's known as a repetition or a rep. Any number of repetitions makes up one set, and any number of sets determines the duration of the workout for that particular muscle. For instance, if you were working on your biceps, you would grasp a dumbbell in each of your hands and curl in towards your shoulder to complete a movement known as a curl. Each time you contract the weight towards your shoulder you are completing one repetition of a bicep curl. A series of repetitions four, six, eight, 10, 12 or even more, would constitute one set.

Ordinarily, you will strive to complete at least three sets of each exercise. For reasons predetermined through carefully controlled experiments, it has been established that a minimum of three sets is what's required to produce desired results.

There is nothing written in stone, however. If you want, you can increase the number of sets or you can increase the number of repetitions in each set you perform. Generally, it's thought that fewer repetitions, with more weight, produces more mass while more repetitions per set, with lighter weights, will produce more definition. This is why we hope to incorporate both strategies in our daily routines.

The rule of thumb for weightlifting, or bodybuilding, is that by steadily increasing the load or the amount of weight you are lifting, over a period of time, you force the muscles to respond by forming new tissue and growing.

For each muscle group you ideally want a variety of exercises, though you won't perform each one during your workout each week. Rather, you choose two or three - possibly even four exercises for each muscle group from among a list of numerous ones known to work well for that particular body part.

Some of these exercises may appear to be very similar, but that's okay. Be assured that each one will work that body part in just a slightly different way so that you eventually get the best all-round results over a period of time. Besides, too much of the same exercise is not only boring and tiresome, but your muscles will actually get so accustomed to the repetition, that they'll eventually level off.

On the other hand, muscles can attain a symbiotic relationship with your brain impulses, over a period of time, which is commonly referred to as muscle memory.

Muscle memory is unique to long-time bodybuilders who can put the sport down for extended periods of time, but have their bodies bounce back to ideal form in a very brief period thanks to this unique phenomenon.

Be patient

Try and remember that big changes aren't going to occur overnight. If you follow the program, these changes will take place relatively quickly, but just don't expect to do it during your first trip to the gym. Don't attempt to push yourself beyond a reasonable maximum for the first few weeks, even if you think you must impress the people around you.

When you step into the gym for the first time, and are overwhelmed at the sight of all those buff bodies, you may be inclined to try and accelerate your routine - possibly thinking you can look like some of these people before the next time you walk through the door. It never happens this way - although it would be nice if it did sometimes.

Start off very easy, and very slowly. Try and remember that you are middle-aged, and that the body you now have has taken 45 or 50 years to get into its current condition. You've also had the affects of gravity working against you all this time, so a lot of your internal organs have probably begun to migrate south, towards your lower abdominal area. Deconstructing the old, and rebuilding the new, is going to take a little while longer than you had hoped, so patience, determination and above all, discipline, are absolutely essential. Remember, this is a lifestyle change.

Weight training has a very direct and relatively rapid affect on self-image and self-esteem. Expect noticeable physical changes to begin occurring with regular training and within a period of weeks. And, when you see these results, you will start feeling a lot more confident and much more in control of your own body.

Although they have good intentions, many people will walk into a gym, try to lift too much weight or work out for too long, maybe won't drink enough water while they are working and the combination of these mistakes will be a bad experience. This leaves their muscles in a state of stiffness, soreness and exhaustion. When this happens, they tend to lose interest while waiting for the soreness to subside. They may never come back for a second workout or they may blame the gym or the routine or anything else for their problems. This is what we want to avoid.

I strongly recommend a two-day-on, day-off method for at least the first three or four weeks of your new fitness lifestyle. On the first day - even if it's the first time in a gym - work your upper body only. On the second day, work only your lower body. Take the third day off to rest your muscles and recover, then start over with your upper body once again.

Each time you work out - whether it's upper body or lower body - you do all the exercise routines designed to work the muscles in that area of your body. For instance, you might do one or two chest exercises, followed by one or two exercises for biceps, triceps, shoulders and back muscles.

For the lower body, only do exercises that work the legs from top to bottom - hamstrings, quadriceps, glutes and calves. Also on this day, work your abdominal muscles, but not too hard. Nothing is worse than having stiff, sore abdominals since it tends to affect every part of your body and may result in a reluctance to go back into the gym until the soreness subsides.

Since there are a great number of exercises for each body part and, since you are only going to be doing one or two per body part during the first phase, you can alternate the exercises. This will do several things for you - it will prevent monotony, and it will give each muscle group a more complete workout over a period of time.

For instance, the chest exercises include bench press, incline bench press, decline bench press, pushups, dumbbell flys, pullovers, cable crossovers and a number of others accomplished through body-specific machinery. Choose just one or two of these for the first workout, then alternate others into your routine over the weeks. This applies not only to the initial phase, but also for the rest of your workouts thereafter.

During this initial phase, pay strict attention to form, so that by the time your muscles are beginning to respond and your energy level is up, you'll be performing each exercise properly, thereby getting the most out of each repetition and benefiting from each workout.

Also, during this time, be certain to spend just a little more time warming up before you hit the weights. Usually I'd recommend eight to10 minutes of cardio exercise, in order to break a sweat and loosen up muscle and tendons. However, in the initial weeks, try 10 to 12 minutes of warm-up, just to be on the safe side, and just to help send a message to your body that things are going to be different in future.

Be certain to complete at least five minutes of stretching between your warm up phase and your workout (see chapter on stretching exercises and techniques). When you are finished working out, do another five minutes or more of stretching before doing your 20-30 minutes of aerobic or cardio training.

Work big upper body muscles, such as the shoulders, a little more carefully than some other areas at first, too. I'd suggest hanging from a chinning bar with your feet off the ground, just to give your shoulders a little extra stretch in the early phase. It's muscles like these that are going to help give your body its new shape: wider at the top, narrower in the middle, and shapelier in the legs.

The same applies for the big leg muscles - glutes, hamstrings, and quadriceps. It's recommended that you choose the leg machines over squats for the first few months, simply because you won't have to worry about balancing a heavy Olympic bar on your shoulders. Your lower back also won't be in any shape to help bear the weight on your shoulders for doing squats.

So, until we've done some work in those primary areas, leave the more advanced exercises to the more experienced people for now.

A common mistake among new weightlifters is to concentrate too much of their energy and attention on obvious areas like the biceps and pectorals. After all, these are the areas that usually impress people more. Nevertheless, there's nothing that looks sillier than having one body part completely out of proportion to the others. Besides, it's actually the tricep muscles that give the upper arm the most definition. Biceps are nice to have, but because they are such a short muscle, they will come up quickly with less work than one might expect. Over time, by working both bicep and tricep muscles equally, you'll have arms like an "anaconda that swallowed a pig"!

Giving your body a complete workout each week, over a period of time, will have an equal effect on all parts of your body, resulting in a symmetrical, more balanced appearance. Working the muscles in the shoulders and back as much as the chest and upper arms will help you stand straighter and taller, and will give you better posture. You're looking for a sleek, well-defined, balanced look in the long run, so stick to your guns (no pun intended, since guns is a word used in reference to bicep muscles).

Chapter 6
The Gym Exercises

Biceps

Chose between dumbbell curls, barbell curls, standing or prone (lying) cable curls, alternate dumbbell curls and a host of other related exercises.

Dumbbell curls: Stand with feet shoulder-width apart, grasp a dumbbell in each hand with the thumbs on the same side as the fingers. Slowly bend the elbow of one arm while lifting the weight towards the shoulder. At the same time, turn your palm inward. When you reach the highest point, hold for a count of two and squeeze the bicep muscle tightly. Inhale before lifting and exhale on the way up, then inhale at the top once more and exhale on the way down. Repeat for the other arm.

Barbell curls: Stand with feet shoulder-width apart, knees slightly bent to take stress off lower back. Again, keep thumbs in line with the fingers while holding bar; don't wrap thumbs around the bar. Bend the elbows of both arms and lift the weight towards the shoulders. Inhale before lifting and exhale during the lift. Pause for a two count at the highest point, inhale and slowly lower weight again while exhaling.

Lying cable curls: Using a straight bar on the bottom fastener of the cable cross-over apparatus, lie face up on the floor with feet braced against base of cable machine and grasp bar firmly with both hands - thumbs aligned with fingers, not wrapped around bar. Curl bar towards shoulders, inhaling before starting and exhaling as you curl. When you reach your shoulder, pause for a two count, then slowly return bar to starting position. Lying on the floor supports the back and takes those muscles out of the movement, so you can use less weight and get better results from this exercise.

Standing cable curls: Using same cable machine, grasp bar and hoist cable towards shoulders. Pause for two count at highest point, then return to starting position.

Preacher bench curls: Rest backs of upper arms against support and grasp barbell with both hands. Inhale and begin raising bar towards shoulders while exhaling. Pause at top for a two count, then return to starting position.

Concentration curls: Sit on a weight bench and place dumbbell between feet. Reach down with one hand and grasp dumbbell. Rest that elbow against the inside of your leg and slowly curl weight towards your shoulder. Pause for a two count, then return to starting position. Do a set of eight to 12 repetitions, then change sides and repeat.

Triceps

Triceps exercises include one- and two-arm cable extensions, overhead cable extensions, dumbbell kickbacks, dips and again, a host of related exercises to choose from on body-specific machinery.

Cable extensions: Grasp the straight bar of the cable crossover machine with the bar in the upper lock position so that your forearms are parallel to the floor in the resting position. Inhale and press down on the bar with your forearms, using only your tricep muscles. When you reach the lowest position hold for a two count then return to the starting or resting position.

For the single arm version, place the handgrip in the upper lock and grasp the handle in one of your hands with your palms facing upward. Your forearm should still be parallel to the floor, but you'll have to stand sideways to position yourself properly. Pull down towards the floor using only your tricep muscle. Pause for a two count, then return to starting position. Do eight to 12 reps, then change hands and repeat.

Dumbbell kickbacks: Hold a dumbbell in one hand and place the opposite knee on the weight bench. Lean over in a kneeling position and place the free hand on the bench, grasping the edge of the bench. With your upper arm parallel to the floor, fully extend your lower arm with the weight hanging freely, then slowly force the weight in a backwards motion until the entire arm is parallel to the floor but behind you. Pause for a two count at the top then slowly lower weight. Do a set of eight to 12 repetitions, change sides and repeat for the other arm.

Overhead cable extensions: Stand with your back to the cable and hold the rope handle in both hands behind your head. With your upper arms parallel to the floor, using your tricep muscles, fully extend the rope handles, pause for a two count, then return to the starting position. Do a set of eight to 12 repetition and three sets.

Arm extensions: Grasp the parallel bars with your hands and hoist yourself off the ground until you are supported by your hands. Slowly bend your elbows and lower yourself until your upper arms reach a point that is roughly parallel to the floor. Hold for a two count then slowly extend your arms, using only your triceps, until your elbows are straight again. Inhale at the top and exhale on the way down. Inhale at the bottom and exhale as your go up. This is an extraordinary exercise for building mass and for giving shape and definition to the triceps.

Back

Back exercises include lower back extensions, seated rowing, cable pulldowns, lat station and, best of all, pullups - wide grip, narrow grip and reverse grip.

Back extensions: Stand in the back extension machine and anchor the backs of your ankles using the soft, foam-rubber pads. Cross your arms in front of your chest and stand straight. Adjust the machine so the support is in your lower abdominal area. Slowly bend forward at the trunk until your head is completely perpendicular, and then extend your lower back to bring your upper body back to the starting position. Do eight to 12 repetitions and three sets.

Seated rowing: Sit with your back upright and your feet firmly against the supports, but with your knees slightly bent to take stress off the lower back. Grasp the handles firmly with the thumb-beside-the-fingers grip rather than the thumb overlapping the handle.

Adjust the weight accordingly. Pull back on the handles until they reach your mid-abdominal area, keeping your back straight and your head and chin up. Pause for a two count, then return to the starting position.

86

Cable pull-downs: Sit with your back straight and your feet firmly on the floor, slightly more than shoulder-width apart. Reach up and grasp handle so that hands are slightly wider than shoulder-width. Adjust weight accordingly. Pull straight down, slowly and deliberately until the bar reaches your upper chest. Pause for a two count, then return to starting position, but maintain tension on the cable until all repetitions are complete.

Lat station: Lay against upper support bench so it is firmly against your chest and your feet are on the base, knees slightly bent to take stress off lower back. Load weights onto front bar or adjust weight rack to suit needs. Reach down and grasp handles firmly with both hands, keeping thumb in align with fingers, not wrapped around the bar. Pull straight back, using your latissimus dorsi muscles as much as possible. Hold for a two count, then slowly return to starting position, keeping tension on the bar all the time.

Pull-ups: Reach up and grasp the bar with palms facing outward slightly more than shoulder width apart. Pull yourself straight up until your chin is above the bar and pause briefly, then lower yourself again. Keep your feet raised off the floor all the time you are performing the exercise. For narrow-grip pull-ups, place your hands on the bar about shoulder-width or slightly closer together, palms facing outward. For reverse-grip pullups, place your hands on the bar, palms facing inward and use a narrow grip. These three exercises work the lower back, late and inner back, but also work shoulders, forearms and almost all the muscles of the upper body. They are difficult to perform, but nothing works faster to shape and contour your upper body.

Shoulders

Shoulder exercises include front dumbbell raises, lateral dumbbell raises, dumbbell salutes, upright rowing, and military press.

Front dumbbell raises: Stand with your feet shoulder-width apart, grasp weights in both hands and hold with palms facing inward, resting against your legs in front of you. Slowly raise your right arm, keeping it straight, palm facing downward, until it is just parallel to the floor. Pause for a two count, then slowly return to the starting position. Repeat for the other arm. Continue until you have completed eight to 12 repetitions for both arms. Do three sets of these. This works the front deltoid muscle most.

Lateral dumbbell raises: Stand as in the front raises, but this time place your arms at your sides, grasping the weights, palms facing inward. Raise both arms at the same time straight out from your sides until they are parallel to the floor. Pause for a two count, then return to starting position. This works the medial deltoid muscle - the shoulder "caps".

Dumbbell salutes: This exercise can be performed alternately, or both arms simultaneously. Stand with feet shoulder-width apart, holding weights in both hands slightly in front of you, palms facing inward, elbows slightly bent. Raise the weights using only your shoulders until the dumbbell is about even with your eyebrow. Pause, and then lower to starting position.

Upright rowing: Stand with feet shoulder-width apart, holding a barbell or the straight bar of the cable machine with hands in the close-grip position. Stand with back straight, face straight ahead. Slowly lift the barbell until it is at eye level, pause, then return to starting position.

Lower Body

The lower body routine will include plenty of choices for each portion of the legs you are going to work out.

The glutes - the big bundle of muscles at the top of the leg, otherwise known as your butt, your buns or your ass - will benefit most from such exercises as standing and lying leg curls. The glutes will also benefit greatly from squat exercises, which also work the quadricep muscles of the upper leg. The quads and glutes will give your leg size, shape and definition but they will also give you the most aggravation when they are sore - and they will become sore, no matter how lightly you work them out at first. Bear with it, because it's only temporary. They are big and require a lot of blood, a lot of energy and a lot of time to train properly.

Leg press: Set yourself comfortably in position with your feet against the platform about shoulder-width apart. Adjust the weight accordingly, but bear in mind that with your back anchored and flat against the support, you'll be able to push more weight than if you were doing squats. About 75-100 pounds on either side is a good place to start and you can move up or down depending on how that goes. Push up on the platform with your legs, disengage the supports, and then slowly lower your legs until your thighs are up against your chest. Pause for a two count then slowly return to the starting position. If you need to spot yourself, place your hands just above your knees and give an extra push as you are extending your legs upward.

Dumbbell/barbell lunges: With a dumbbell in either hand, place your feet slightly apart and face forward, head up. Extend your right foot a good pace forward and bend at the knee until your thigh is parallel to the floor. Keep the other foot stationary and as you move forward stretch the back leg out until you feel a slight pull. Return to the starting position and change sides.

With the barbell, hoist it straight over your head, and then lower it until the bar is resting comfortably atop your shoulders (not on the back of your neck). Perform the same procedure as with the dumbbells.

Front squats: Grasp a barbell in both hands, palms forward, and curl it up to your shoulders. Hold it here, pressed firmly against your upper chest, then bend at the knees and slowly lower yourself until your thighs are parallel to the floor. Loosen your hips when you do this and make certain your knees are pointing outwards. Pause at the bottom, then slowly return to the starting position, keeping your back straight and your head forward. Use a very light weight at first until you become comfortable with this exercise.

Leg extensions: Sit in the leg extension machine and adjust the back support so you are comfortable. Place your hands on the handles at your sides and put your ankles behind the foam pads. Using your quadricep muscles, raise your ankles until they are parallel to the floor, pause for a two-count, then return slowly to the starting position. This exercise will split the quadricep muscle just above the knee and give it thickness and definition.

Standing/lying hamstring curls: Lay face-down on the hamstring machine, grasp the handles firmly for support, look straight ahead and place the backs of your ankles under the foam pads. Adjust weight to suit your needs, but you'll likely want to begin with a very light weight - 20 pounds or so. Slowly curl the backs of your ankles towards your buttocks until they meet, hold for a two-count, and then slowly return to the starting position. However, stop just short of letting the cable slack off - keeping tension on the cable all the time. Repeat for eight to 12 reps and three sets.

For the standing variation, position yourself comfortably and place the backs of your ankles in front of the foam pads. Bend your right knee and curl the pad toward your buttock until the two meet. Hold for a two count, and then slowly return to the starting position. Repeat for the other leg.

Calf raises on leg press: Sit in the leg press as though you were going to work your quads, but position your feet so that only the portion from the balls of the feet forward at making contact with the sled platform. Extend your feet as though you were standing on your tip-toes and pause at the top for a two-count, then return to the starting position. Maintaining tension on the sled during the entire set will benefit you more. Point your toes inward for one set, parallel to each other for another set, and for the third set point the toes outward. This way, you work all parts of the calf muscles, giving them definition as well as size.

A word about the calves: The calf muscles are similar to the abdominals in that they respond best when tension is kept on them all the time. Do your calf exercises quickly, maintaining tension at all times for better response.

Donkey calf raises: This can be performed with a donkey calf machine or with your partner sitting on your back, down around your hips. Bend at the trunk until your upper body is parallel to the floor and brace yourself against the wall or hold on to a piece of equipment. With your feet on a step and your heels hanging over the edge, raise yourself using only your calf muscles. When you get to the top, pause for a two count, then return to a position slightly lower than where you began - this helps to stretch the calf muscles.

Quads will also benefit as well as aerobic activity such as stop and start sprints, tennis, soccer and skating - both inline and ice varieties.

The hamstrings will also benefit from standing and lying leg curls, while the calves can be built up from exercises such as one and two-legged donkey raises (standing with the balls of the foot, or feet, on the edge of a step and raising oneself up until the calf muscle is fully flexed).

Again, there are also a host of related exercises available on body-specific machinery designed for the lower body and almost any gymnasium has these machines.

From time to time, somebody attempts to reinvent the wheel when it comes to exercise routines. You've probably seen infomercials and magazine advertisements for these products, each supposedly designed to do in a matter of minutes, what should take hours in a gym. This equipment seldom if ever works the way is was intended. More often than not it doesn't work at all. The best policy is to do it the way it has always been done. When you finally arrive at your destination - a buff and lean body - feel free to purchase any number of simple exercise machines that could supplement your workouts or allow you to maintain your physique without having to go into the gym if you like. For now, stick to the basics.

Abdominal muscle workouts are numerous and varied, perhaps more so than any other body area since there are a number of muscle groups that make up the complex muscular system which holds our organs inside our abdominal cavities.

More than any other body area, numerous pieces of machinery and specialty apparatus have been designed specifically to target the abdominals. The reason for this is simple. This area, more than any other, stands as a measure of how fit or how fat any particular person may be. If you've got a flabby belly, you can run, but you can't hide forever. Sooner or later there will be that inevitable trip to the beach, or maybe a winter vacation to some sunny climate. A flat stomach, with well-defined abdominal muscles, makes a man sleek and sexy. What's more, it does more than anything else to give one good posture.

Every gym these days has at least one or two machines designed specifically for the abs. If these aren't available, don't be concerned. After all, even machines designed to target such a crucial, specific area won't work unless you make them work.

Crunches, leg lifts, hanging leg lifts, arm-knee crossovers and a host of other related exercises will do the job just as well. Better, in fact.

Unlike other body parts, the abdominal workout doesn't require weights. Nevertheless, you may still come across a lot of bodybuilders who will add weight to their ab routines in an effort to make those muscles stand out more. Most of what is required to have good abs is the ability to pay strict attention to your diet - that and plenty of repetitious action in this area.

Before you go spending upwards of an hour each day trying to make your abdominals stand out from that sagging, flabby belly, remember that proper nutrition and thermogenics, or fat-burning, brought about by additional muscle mass is necessary in order for your abs to show. If you find you've been working them hard, but they still don't show through the skin, the reason is that layer of fat covering them. Chances are, they are hard and ripped under those layers of subcutaneous fat, but they just aren't visible at this time.

And you can't spot reduce this area - without liposuction, that is.

A new and healthy eating routine, as outlined here, combined with a steady exercise program in the gym along with aerobic training three or four times a week will eventually result in well-defined abdominal muscles. They aren't going to appear overnight and they aren't going to appear at all unless you follow the nutritional guidelines faithfully and have some discipline. Keep this thought in mind, though: Once you can see your abdominals, you'll know the rest of your body is lean and fit as well. Now there's something you can really strive to attain.

Proper form is essential

The key to getting the most from each workout and to getting the most from your time in the gym is to get into the habit of practising proper form at all times. Perform each exercise the way it was intended, without cheating. A few well-performed repetitions are more beneficial than dozens of cheaters.

Don't try to lift more weight than is possible to comfortably complete a set of eight to 12 repetitions - for any muscle group. If you think you can do 120 pounds, try 80 or 90 to start with, because it's probably heavier than it looks. Also, by lifting more weight than you should be, you'll end up using muscles that you don't want to use when you are keying on a specific body part.

More weight will also cause you to perform the exercise in a herky, jerky manner that could result in an injury to that muscle and/or your back. To make matters worse, you'll end up dropping the weight or having it come crashing down which will create an embarrassing situation for you. At this point you probably would just as soon draw as little attention to yourself as possible during your first few visits - at least until you get your confidence built up, that is.

Your prime concern, in the early stages, is to preserve the integrity of your back. We don't want to damage any vertebrates, nor do we want to end up with torn back muscles or something equally nasty and hurtful. Once we get our backs into shape, along with the rest of the body, we can step up the program a bit more and incorporate some of those free-weight exercises in which the back comes into play more often. In the meantime, be aware of your back and keep a safe workout in mind.

In some specific exercises, such as bicep curls, a lot of people will end up using their back muscles as much or more so than the biceps in order to curl more weight than they should be lifting. If you end up doing this, you won't be doing your biceps any favours and you could also end up with that injury thing happening.

The way to avoid this pitfall is to lie on your back and use the cable crossover apparatus to perform your bicep curls. Brace your feet against the base and attach a straight bar to the lowest end of the cable machine. In a prone position, curl the bar up to your shoulders and hold for a one count, then slowly return to the downward position.

By performing bicep curls in this manner, you won't be using your back to lift the weight and won't be cheating. You'll end up with better bicep gains over the long run because the exercise concentrates all the effort into those muscles alone.

Ditto for abdominal exercises. Don't bother with setups. I know these were the standard procedure for abdominal work way back when, but they don't work worth a hoot for your stomach muscles. They will work your hip flexor muscles, but not your abs. Even if you can do a thousand situps, it isn't going to give you washboard abdominals or anything even close to this affect.

Stick to the exercises described earlier - crunches, leg raises, hanging leg raises and so on, they work faster and better, especially if you can get "in the zone" during the early repetitions so that when you max out at 15 or 20 reps, your stomach is hurting like crazy.

During the execution of any exercise, try and relax the muscles which are not being used to perform that particular exercise. This includes your face. Grimacing and making horrid faces won't make the repetition any easier and it forces extra blood into that region when it could be better used in another part of the body.

Doing leg squats is another exercise that is of great benefit to your lower body, but which can cause damage to your upper body, especially your back, if you don't have the proper form. Unless you have spent some time in a gym up to this point, or unless you are already in fairly decent condition, I wouldn't recommend squats until such time as you are feeling more fit and confident in your level of fitness.

However, lower body and leg workouts are important and essential to getting a balanced look so instead of squats, try the leg press machine, or perhaps the hack squat machines. These machines have you lying on your back - therefore fully supported - with your feet braced against a weight sled. This not only allows you to concentrate on the quadricep muscles and glutes, but also saves you from having to balance a heavy bar across your shoulders, thus eliminating the chance of hurting your back through improper lifting.

Eventually you will want to incorporate leg squats into your weekly fitness regime. When you do, remember that Instead of thinking the weight is on your shoulders, imagine it is below your feet, just as it is in the leg press machine. When you lift, imagine you are pushing your feet through the floor rather than pushing the weight on your shoulders. You'll be surprised at what a difference it makes and how much easier the exercise will seem.

Remember also that squats involve the biggest muscles in the body, so it is going to require a lot of energy and a lot of intensity.

The Weekly Gymnasium Routine

Following is a day-by-day, week-by-week example of what you should be doing now in order to put these principles of good nutrition and good fitness into play. There is plenty of variation in the exercises and some variation from week-to-week. Once you get familiar with this routine, try incorporating some addition exercises into the program.

First Week

Day 1: Upper Body

dumbbell bicep curls
tricep cable extensions
bench press
cable pulldowns (back)
military press (shoulders)
crunches (abdominals)

* Be sure you use very light weights for each of these exercises. Do at least eight to 10 repetitions for each exercise and at least three sets. Don't forget to warm up and stretch before starting,

and don't forget to do at least 20 minutes of cardio, followed by another stretching session, when you are finished.

Incidentally, be sure to do all the exercises for any particular body part before moving on to another body part. Don't mix exercises for various body parts. Do all the bicep exercises in consecutive order - whatever order you choose. Then move on to another body part and do all the exercises which are geared for that body part. Always do this, it works more efficiently because then the blood doesn't have to reroute to a different body part in the middle of an exercise, then reroute itself back to the original part and so on.

Day 2: Lower Body

leg press
lying cable hamstring curls
cable leg extensions
calf raises

*As with day one, be sure to warm up and stretch - particularly the lower body areas - before your workout. Again, use light weights for everything - say 50 per cent of your body weight for the leg press, and a reasonable amount for all other machines. Do your cardio and stretch afterwards.

Day 3: Rest

Day 4: Upper Body

*Repeat all the exercises you did on day one, using the same amount of weight for each exercise. Do the same number of reps and perform the same number of sets.

Day 5: Lower Body

*Repeat day two lower body exercises, again using same weights, same reps and same sets. Do warm-up and stretch before as well as cardio and stretching afterward.

Second Week

Day 1: Upper Body

* Repeat all exercises you performed for upper body during the first week but add a minimum of 10 per cent and a maximum of 15 per cent to all weight totals. Add two reps to each set but perform the same number of sets. Don't forget to warm up and stretch and do cardio and stretch afterward.

Day 2: Lower Body

*As with the upper body routine, perform same lower body routines as in week one but again, add 10 per cent to weight totals and a maximum of 15 per cent. Add two reps to each set but perform the same number of sets. Don't forget to warm up and stretch and do cardio and stretch afterward.

Day 3: Rest

Day 4: Upper Body

*Repeat day 1 including warm up and cardio and all stretching.

Day 5: Lower Body

*Repeat day 2 including warm up and cardio and all stretching.

Third Week

Day 1: Upper Body

dumbbell bicep curls
dumbbell hammer curls
tricep kick backs
bench press
dumbbell flys
cable pulldowns (back)

Seated rowing (back)
military press (shoulders)
crunches (abdominals)
bicycle crunches (elbows to opposite knees)

* Increase weight again by as much as 10 per cent on all the exercises you were previously doing. However, go with minimal weight on the new exercises we've introduced at this point. Do warm up, stretching, cardio afterwards.

Day 2: Lower Body

Dumbbell lunges
leg press
leg extensions
lying hamstring curls
calf raises on leg press machine

* Again, as in the upper body work this week, increase the weight slightly - perhaps as much as 10 per cent if you are feeling up to it. If not, don't rush it and go back to whatever weight you were formerly using. Use minimal weight for new exercises. Don't forget warm-up before, stretch and cardio afterward.

Day 3: Rest

Day 4: Upper Body

Incline bench press
dumbbell flys
military press
dumbbell salutes
seated rowing
back extensions (lower back)
dumbbell kickbacks

* Use the same weights you were using on Day 1 upper body exercises. Again, warm up, stretch, cardio.

Day 5: Lower Body

Repeat all exercises you performed on Day 2 this week, using the same amount of weight. Warm up, stretch, cardio.

Fourth Week

Day 1: Upper Body

dumbbell hammer curls
barbell bicep curls
bench press
decline press
tricep cable extensions
tricep dumbbell kickbacks
military press
dumbbell salutes
reverse crunches
bicycle crunches

* Keep the same amount of weight on all exercises but increase the number of repetitions in each set. Do at least three sets for each exercise except the abdominal crunches, which should have sets of at least 20 reps.

Day 2: Lower Body

leg press
barbell lunges
lying cable hamstring curls
leg extensions
calf raises

* Bump up the amount of weight slightly once more for all these exercises and don't forget to do your warm up, stretch and cardio afterward.

Day 3: Rest

Day 4: Upper Body

dumbbell hammer curls
barbell bicep curls
incline bench press
pec deck
tricep cable extensions
tricep dumbbell kickbacks
military press
dumbbell salutes
reverse crunches
bicycle crunches

* Keep the same amount of weight on all exercises, but increase the number of repetitions in each set. Do at least three sets for each exercise except the abdominal crunches, which should have sets of at least 20 reps.

Day 5: Lower Body

leg press
barbell lunges
lying cable hamstring curls
leg extensions
calf raises

* Bump up the amount of weight slightly once more for all the exercises.

Fifth week

Day 1: cardio, stretching and abdominal work

Day 2: rest

Day 3: cardio, stretching and abs

Day 4: rest

Day 5: Cardio, stretching and abdominals

Day 6: rest

At this point, there is going to be a major shift in the way we work our muscles. We are going to move to a system whereby we work each muscle just once a week. The first four weeks of training have by now forced your muscles to adjust to a regular schedule of working against continually increasing resistance. Meanwhile, the week off in week 5 will give you some much-needed time for rest and recovery before we embark on the second and more concentrated phase of our body shaping routine.

While we worked at steadily increasing the amount of weight we were using each week through the first weeks, now we will be increasing the weight load during each workout.

Begin with a light set for each exercise and do at least 12 repetitions. For the second set, add some weight - whatever you are comfortable with, but not a great deal - and perform 10 repetitions. For the third set, increase the amount of weight once more and perform eight reps. Set four will be more weight and six reps while the fifth set will see yet another weight increase and only four repetitions. Finish each exercise by dropping the amount of weight to what you used in the first set - or even lighter - and perform repetitions to failure - meaning you keep doing reps until you can't do any more.

Use this system for each exercise, with the exception of your abdominal workouts which will now take place three times each week.

Sixth Week

Day 1: chest, triceps and abdominals

dumbbell flys
bench press
decline bench
cable tricep extensions
dumbbell kickbacks
hanging leg raises
reverse crunches

* Do at least 20 repetitions and three sets each for the abdominals exercises. Don't forget to warm up, stretch and do cardio afterward.

Day 2: Legs

Light squats
leg press
seated leg extensions
Hamstring curls - standing and lying variations
leg press calf raises
donkey calf raises

*Finish your leg routine with this additional exercise: crouch as low to the floor as possible, then spring into the air as high as possible - as though you are performing a standing vertical jump. Continue doing these for 30 straight seconds (it's much harder than you might think). Wait one minute and do another 30-second set. Wait another minute, and then do a third and final 30-second set. Be sure to warm up before your daily routine, but don't bother with the cardio on leg day.

Day 3: Rest

Day 4: Back, forearms and abdominals

Seated rowing
cable pulldowns
wide-grip chin ups (as many as possible, and three sets)
back extensions
reverse curls (forearms)
wrist curls
hanging leg-raises
reverse crunches
side trunk bends

*Warm up and stretch before beginning the day and do 20-30 minutes of cardio afterward.

Day 5: biceps, shoulders, abdominals

Lying cable curls
dumbbell concentration curls
dumbbell hammer curls
dumbbell salutes
standing barbell rowing
military press
bicycle crunches (three sets of 30 - 40 reps)
Roman chair crunches

*The lying cable curls are the major difference now. Nothing builds your biceps quicker than this exercise, which isolates the bicep while taking your back and all the other muscles out of the equation. The hammer curls work the forearms as well as the bicep but help to give your biceps sharper peaks. Anytime you grip a barbell or dumbbell, keep your thumbs behind the bar, not wrapped around. This may take a little getting used to but it makes for a stronger grip in the long run and works the muscles your are targeting better.

Day 6: rest

Day 7: rest

Repeat

Breathe properly

Proper breathing is also essential to get the most benefit from your repetitions. Inhale before lifting, exhale while lifting, and then inhale again while lowering the weight. Try not to hold your breath and try not to tense other muscles - such as those in your face - while performing the exercise. Creating tension in body areas other than the one you are exercising will take away energy you need to perform that exercise, plus in will needlessly raise your blood pressure.

Try and keep an accurate daily journal, at least for the first six to eight weeks, if you are just going into the gym for the first time or for the first time in a long time. This way, you can keep better track of your progress. It also helps you keep track of the exercises you've performed for each body part, the weights you've used, the number of sets and the number of reps.

Eventually you'll likely be able to keep track of these things just as easily in your head although some people like to keep a daily workout journal all the time. Whatever works best for you is the thing to do in this case.

Chapter 7
Free Weights or Machines?

Most anyone who enters a gym for the first time is going to be confronted with a variety of options. Do you use free weights - barbells and dumbbells - or do you use the variable resistance machines with their cables and pulleys, cams and levers?

Experienced body builders prefer free weights, since they achieve their most notable gains by use of these. This is mainly because free weights not only allow you to train the target muscle group, but they engage other muscles that assist in the work. Once they are conditioned, these assisting - or synergistic - muscles help the body builder to increase the weight used in training the target muscles which helps to stimulate the most growth in the muscle fibres.

Those fancy machines, on the other hand, are designed to work specific muscles in nearly complete isolation from the assisting muscles. For this reason, you can't use as much weight on these machines as you might be able to with free weights.

Machines can only be adjusted for a certain range of height and physique, so if you happen to be six feet, four inches, chances are pretty slim that you'll be fitting comfortably into machines that were designed with men of average height in mind.

In defense of free weights, it should be noted that they could help to improve your balance and coordination more than the variable resistance machines, since you must always control and balance the weights yourself, without the aid of the machine.

However, whether you choose to use free weights exclusively or not, you'll still be required to make use of standard machines such as leg extension machines, leg curl machines, lat machines and other devices that work extremely well in shaping your body.

The only other advice here is that when looking for a gymnasium; don't simply look at the quantity and quality of the equipment and free weights available. Also take a close look at cleanliness, neatness and the condition of the equipment. All the fancy machines in the world are no good to anyone if they are always out of order. This can also be very frustrating and can make you second-guess your choice of gym once your membership dues are paid.

Be certain there is enough room around individual workstations and that there are a number of the same type of station in that particular gym. A lot of compact gyms have plenty of members, but the workstations are packed closely together. This often doesn't leave enough room for you to comfortably work out without running into someone working near you at some other exercise. Similarly, if there is only one workout station for exercises such as squats, bench press and so on, you'll end up waiting for that station to be freed up so you can workout.

Just about any gym you find these days is filled to overflowing with high-quality equipment. In some cases it may even be filled with specialty machines that work each individual muscle group efficiently and properly. If the gym you choose is one of these, so much the better. If not, don't despair. In spite of the way these machines operate, it doesn't do anything else but exercise the muscle and you can do that with any free weights just as easily and in most cases, just as effectively. Besides, the key here is not necessarily to become another Arnold Schwarzenegger, only to get toned and fit... and maybe just a little buff in the process.

Of course, if getting really buff has always been your passion, once you reach a certain point in this program you can take it as far as you wish. What's more, I'll also show you how to work muscle groups and body areas effectively and efficiently without the use of those machines I mentioned earlier.

If you can't get to a gym you can improvise effectively if you can at least arrange to have a chinning bar in a doorway inside your home. Or, you can exercise effectively outdoors, using equipment provided free of charge in playgrounds and public parks. I stayed in top form for more than five years using only an outdoor public park and doing nothing more than chinups, pushups and dips along with some home abdominal work. The point is, even if your gym burns down, or if you should suddenly find yourself confined to your home, or even if you've been locked out of your house, there is a way to a full-body fitness routine that can put you in the best shape of your life.

And just a word or two about the people you may encounter in a gymnasium. Ideally, they'll be friendly, cooperative and non-judgmental, but don't count on it. Too often people are intimidated by attitudes within the gym. For reasons unbeknownst to most folks, some of the more brain-dead bodybuilders like to give the impression they were born that way or that the equipment "belongs" to them. Ignore these people and go about your routine as though you have horse blinders on. Even if it makes you feel a little uncomfortable at first, you'll soon become confident and oblivious of the steroid monsters and obsessive-compulsives who inhabit some gyms.

Flexibility

Flexibility is the term we use to describe the ability of the joints to move through their natural range of motion. By being flexible and maintaining a high degree of flexibility, we can reduce the risk of sports-related injuries while at the same time improving our balance, posture and athletic performance.

We can and should do a great deal to retain and even improve our flexibility as we age since maintaining flexibility as the years go by will help you move like a young man. The natural aging process and inactivity are the worst enemies of our flexibility. A sedentary lifestyle will result in the loss of elasticity in the connective tissue and shortening of the muscles associated with the joints. If you are stiff and sore and have very little flexibility because of a lifetime of inactivity, a daily series of stretching exercises will overcome this problem.

Eventually, if you are stretching daily, you will be able to do almost anything a child can do where acts of flexibility are concerned. Even five minutes of stretching done three or four ties a week will help keep you loose.

Between sets, get into the habit of doing additional stretching of the body part you are working on that day. Every little bit helps in the battle to regain and maintain your flexibility. If you stretch after a workout or after an aerobic conditioning session, when your muscles and tendons are warm, you'll get the most benefit.

If you have trouble stretching, or have been trying for some time with limited results, try getting a book on stretching from your library or try taking a yoga course. You may also enroll in a stretch and strength class at your local fitness club or even invest in a video designed specifically for stretching.

Some people are naturally more flexible than others, but if you've done everything right and you're in good shape, you should be able to get your legs behind your head. If you can't, keep working at it.

What's more, keeping the muscles of your legs and back flexible can help prevent back pain and can aid in keeping the discs between the vertebrae supple and in a healthy condition.

A good stretching exercise for the lower back and upper hamstrings is to cross your legs at the ankle, while standing, then slowly bend at the waist while reaching down with your arms until your hands won't go any further. Hold this position for a count of 30 seconds, then slowly come back to an upright position and repeat, only this time cross your legs in the opposite direction. Do this two or three times a week until you are able to reach the floor with your fingers, then until you can place your palms flat on the floor. It'll happen, you just have to give it a little time and keep at it.

Another excellent stretch for the lower back is one where you lay flat on the floor, face-down, with your hands palms-down on the floor beside your shoulders, as though you are going to do a pushup. With your body from the waist down still flat on the floor, raise your upper body slightly, then slowly raise it as high as possible on your hands until your feel it stretching your lower back. Hold at this point and count slowly to 30, then raise yourself a little higher and count to 30 once more. Continue doing this until you can eventually extend your arms fully while still keeping your lower body flat on the floor.

Lying on your back, bring your legs slowly up while at the same time bending your knees. At the same time, reach down with your

108

hands and place them on your shins or ankles and draw your legs tightly into your chest in a fetal position. Hold this position for the count of 30, then slowly return to the lying position and repeat two or three times. You can also do this same stretch with just one leg at a time.

Eventually, work your way up to the ultimate stretch of the lower back and trunk area: lie flat on your back, then raise both your legs and your arms, keeping both straight with knees and elbows locked, until your feet and hands meet above you and your face is looking directly at your crotch. Hold this for a count of 30 as well.

Before working out and after you've completed your eight to 10 minutes of cardio warm up, spend at least three to five minutes stretching every area of your body that you can think of. Grasp your ankles and pull your leg gently up to your buttocks and hold it for a count of up to 30 seconds, then do the same thing with the other leg. Be sure you grasp your foot by the ankle, not by the top of your toes.

Stretch your arms into the air above your head and reach as high as possible for another count of 30 seconds. Then, bend them one at a time at the elbow while reaching across with the other hand and grabbing hold of the opposite elbow. Gently pull on that elbow to give your shoulders, triceps and upper back a little more of a stretch. Hold this for a count of 30 as well, then trade sides and do the same thing with the other arm.

Another excellent stretch is one where you put both hands behind your back, lock your fingers together, and then extend your arms until your elbows are strait. Hold this position for a count of 30 seconds, then slowly bend at the waist, while still maintaining the behind-the-back positioning of the arms and try to get your head down as far as it will go. At the same time, raise your arms in a backward motion until they are straight up in the air while your head is pointing at the floor. Again, hold this position for a count of 30, or at least as long as you can manage. A major stretch like this will be somewhat uncomfortable at first, depending on how long it has been since you stretched, and how flexible you are in the first place.

If you are planning to work your shoulder and/or triceps on that particular day, you might want to try an additional stretching exercise using the inside of the door jam. Stand up close to the door jam and reach your hand above your head and place the palm of your hand flat against the inside door jam. Then slowly move sideways a little closer towards the jam until your flank is butted up against it and your arm, with the palm against the jam, is extended all the way to a perpendicular position. Hold for thirty seconds, then repeat, and then do the same thing on the other side.

An excellent stretch for the shoulders and upper back is one you can perform inside any doorway - in the gym, in the office or especially at home. Stand right inside the doorway and reach up to the door sill with both hands and place your palms against the sill in the same direction your are facing. Then, gently lean your body forward ever so slightly until your feel a good stretch in your shoulders and back and hold this for a count of 30. Stand on your toes, if necessary.

There are plenty of other good stretching exercises your can incorporate but be sure your find at least one for each area of your body and do it; three-to-five times a week, especially on days when you are in the gym.

If you want to accelerate the process of getting into shape and toning your body, do a good five-to-10-minute stretch each morning upon rising. Your aging body is going to resist this newfound regimen for a little while, but eventually will become accustom to the new challenge. Keep doing this and you'll never feel still and sore when you get out of bed any more. Wouldn't that alone be worth the effort?

Your enemies

The worst enemies of the human body, particularly the abdominal area in men, is the simple carbohydrate and the "trans-fatty acids" found in fast food, junk food, and chocolate.

In a woman, fat is stored on the hips and the breasts more than any other area, while on men, fat is stored on the back and the abdomen. If you have the inclination, have a test to determine the amount of body fat you are currently carrying. The average for a man is about 17-24 per cent, while the average for a woman is slightly higher.

Don't expect to see abdominal muscles until you get down below 15 per cent body fat on a regular basis. Those pictures you've seen of bodybuilders with the incredible abdominals is a result of a body-fat percentage of only three to five per cent, and they can only maintain this for a day or two, at most, before they become drastically sick. I would never recommend a body-fat percentage lower than eight per cent for anyone for health reasons. If you even reach 10 per cent, you'll be, as they say, "ripped to shreds" by comparison to the average guy walking the streets. A realistic goal is 10-to-12 percent, and that can easily be reach by following the diet and nutritional information you're find here.

Incidentally, fat testing can be done in a number of ways. One of the simplest and quickest ways is with a pair of "fat calipers," which measure the thickness of certain areas of the body - abdomen, back, arms legs, etc. From these measurements, a fairly accurate idea of body fat content can be calculated, but it will only be within a percent or two of complete accuracy.

A more exact method of measurement is the fat dunk tank, in which you submerge yourself in a tank of water. Depending on the amount of water that is displaced, according to your weight, your body fat content can be more precisely determined.

Sometimes it's a good idea to get a body fat measurement from the start of your program so you can gradually see just how much difference diet, nutrition and fitness are making on the physical makeup of your body. It can also show you just how far you've let yourself go over the years though this is usually the kind of news nobody wants to hear about.

Chapter 9
Aerobics And Cardio Conditioning

In addition to the gym routines, plan to incorporate some sort of aerobic activity into your weekly fitness program by performing some type of continuous exercise that will get your heart rate up to about 80 per cent of its maximum for 20 minutes or longer. This is not just important; it's pivotal, if you hope to accomplish what we've laid out here. Twenty to forty minutes, three or four times a week is necessary whether it be on a treadmill, a bicycle, stationary bike, stairstepper, jogging, walking, swimming or what have you. Be certain you include aerobics in your lifestyle.

Increasing the aerobic capacity of the lungs means they will be able to carry more oxygen while the benefits to the circulatory system means the blood will better be able to carry this oxygen, along with nutrients, to the muscles to make them grow faster. At the same time, it will allow the body to excrete toxins and carbon dioxide more efficiently.

It's also a good idea to vary your aerobic workout just like you do with your gym workouts and for the same reasons. There are even more benefits to this variation, however. Your legs will benefit even more from cycling, playing tennis or soccer and from skating. Besides, you can't spend your whole life indoors so exercise such as cycling, swimming and, in particular, inline skating, allow you to explore the great outdoors. What's more, learning to dodge traffic and deal with angry motorists will open a whole new world to most people.

The least advisable exercise for anyone at this stage of life is to take up running or jogging. Regardless of what you may have heard and what you've seen, the aerobic benefits from this type of exercise are outweighed by the negative affects all that pounding on asphalt will have on your joints. The hip joints, knees and ankles will take a tremendous beating, even if you buy the most expensive running shoes in the world. The other aerobic exercises I've already mentioned will give you a superior cardio workout with far less stress on the joints.

However, if you are already a runner and have enjoyed this form of exercise, more power to you. If that's all you are doing, take a closer look at the people around you who are doing the same thing. Are they healthy looking, or do they appear emaciated? Do you want to look like a long-distance runner, or do you want to look a little more like Sylvester Stalone in Rocky II?

How are your joints feeling right now? Your hips? Your Knees? Your ankles? Have you taken the time to study the long-term affects of running on your body?

Keep in mind that wind sprints or playing a game of ice hockey is not necessarily an aerobic activity. These forms of extremely vigorous exercise - short bursts of energy over brief periods, followed by a period of rest - are actually what are known as anaerobic activity. These have a far different affect on your body than do aerobic workouts.

If you elevate your heart rate too much, say more than 200 beats per minute, which is entirely possible if you are doing either of the aforementioned activities, you go into an anaerobic state, during which time your body will deplete its stores of glycogen (Glucose molecules hooked together in long chains and stored in the liver and muscles as energy reserves). The body works in mysterious ways. In a situation like this, it will opt to conserve its stores of fat and instead begin burning lean muscle tissue as an energy source. The result is a situation in which you are doing just the opposite of what you set out to do. Instead of burning fat, you will be burning muscle. Climbing the stairs of the CN Tower in Toronto would be another example of an anaerobic workout.

By contrast, an aerobic workout should only take your heart rate up to 115-140 beats per minute, perhaps even a little less, depending on your age and your level of fitness at the time. However, you must target the 80 per cent of maximum heart rate area. This will put your body into an aerobic state at which time it begins using up its stores of fat as an energy source once it has depleted its stores of glycogen in the muscles and in the liver.

The beauty of aerobics is that your body will often remain in an aerobic state for as much as an hour or longer after you finish your workout.

If you plan to incorporate your aerobics into your gym workout, wait until after you have done your gym workout before climbing on the aerobic equipment. This combination of weight training and aerobics elevates the production of testosterone while building lean muscle mass and burning fat at the same time. It's an unbeatable combination that has been proven highly effective time and again.

Avoid Overtraining

To get the most from your muscles in the least amount of time requires that you don't overwork them. Sounds odd, but it's true. Overtraining is a common pitfall among even the most serious and dedicated of bodybuilders. Overtraining - training too hard, for too long a period of time or too often during the same week, will result in less dynamic muscle tone and won't get you the kind of gains you can achieve by doing just the right amount of training.

The key is to work each muscle once each week, with the exception of the abs, which almost always need a little more work. Nevertheless, if you want to keep everything to a simple once-a-week routine, work your abdominals once weekly as well.

The reason we work our muscles only once a week is that rest and recovery time is every bit as important as the exercise itself if you want them to grow. Accumulating quality muscle and muscle tone takes some time and the result is a buffer, better-looking body.

The rest and recovery period is essential, however. When we work out a muscle, such as the biceps, the act of lifting the weight actually tears the muscle fibres ever so slightly. During rest and recovery phase, the body heals this tear and the new muscle tissue it forms to heal that tear adds to the overall size of the muscle itself. It's not the act of lifting the weight that creates the additional muscle size, but the repair and recovery that creates the additional girth.

Try some variation

Too much of the same thing gets downright boring and if you get bored of working out, chances are you may decide to start missing the odd workout. Eventually this lethargic attitude could permeate your entire being and we don't want to risk that happening.

So, try a little variation - not only in your workout routines, but also in your aerobic activity and your weekend and vacation activity.

Climb on your bicycle occasionally, if you don't already do this. Get out ice skating once in a while during winter months, and try and get into a pool and swim some lengths at least a few times a month. A brisk walk every other day wouldn't hurt and would actually aid in digestion and the peristaltic action of the stomach and intestines.

If you play golf, by all means don't stop and try to maintain other weekly recreational activities as well if you are already actively pursuing these interests - handball, squash, racquetball, tennis, curling, rock-climbing, baseball and the like. The more variation you put your body through, the more challenges you throw at it, the more it will respond, even if you've been away from most of these activities for years or even decades.

In the gym, incorporate new and innovative ways to workout the same muscles you might have been working on for months. Add a new exercise here, drop an old one there, shock the muscles and watch them respond.

Chapter 10
The Home Gym

Even if you have a gym membership, sometimes you can't get there and occasionally you might want to take a few weeks or a month-long hiatus from the gym atmosphere. This is allowable and actually recommended once a year or so. This can keep you toned and muscular while you recharge your batteries and prepare yourself mentally to get back to a healthy gym workout routine. If you happen to live in a rural area or so far out in the 'burbs that there is no gymnasium, then working out at home can be a viable alternative, provided you put the same kind of effort into your workouts and exercise the same discipline in your eating habits and your nutritional goals.

All you really need for a decent home gym is a pair of dumbbells - about 20 lbs apiece, although once you get accustomed to working with this weight you may want to purchase a slightly heavier set. You may also find a workout bench handy though this is optional since a coffee table will do if nothing else is available. You can also lay an ironing board (legs folded up) between two chairs to fashion yourself a bench as well. A pair of ankle weights are also handy to have and can really add to the intensity of your home workout for areas such as the buttocks, hamstrings, lower back and inner thighs.

Since you are going to be working out at home, taking a day of rest between each workout should be no problem and this will promote optimum muscle growth while allowing plenty of time for the all-important rest and repair phase. Just as in the gym, break your workout into body areas - biceps and chest one day, lower body and abdominals another day, triceps and back another day, shoulders and abdominals another day. These are only suggested routines; your own can vary depending on your own time frame and your own preference.

If you are working out at home, don't neglect your eight- to 10-minute warm-up and your five minutes of stretching before you begin. Afterward, don't forget about your cardio routine - even if this means skating around the neighbourhood on inline roller skates, riding your bicycle or mountain bike or climbing on a stationary bike, treadmill or stairstepper, provided you have these in your home.

Here are the suggested exercises for the various body areas:

Lower Body: buttocks, hamstrings, lower back and inner thighs: An exercise called opposite extensions works all these muscle areas quite well. After you do them without weights for a few weeks, add your ankle and/or wrist weights to increase the load and work everything that much harder for a little growth in these areas.

Lie face down with your forehead resting on your left hand and your legs straight - toes pointed out, heels together. Tighten your abdominal muscles and try to create a space between your stomach and the floor.

Lift and extend your right arm forward as you squeeze your buttocks muscle and at the same time, lift and extend your left leg back. Don't lift your limbs very high, only about a foot or so off the floor. Hold the extension for a count of three, then slowly lower your limbs to the floor and repeat. When you've done a set of eight to 12 repetitions, change sides and do the opposite limbs for the same number of repetitions. Do at least three sets for each side.

Buttocks, quadriceps and hamstrings: An exercise known as the bench lunge works these muscle groups effectively. Again, once you have mastered the technique and have gone several weeks, hold your dumbbells in your hands to increase the load on these muscles. Combined with an aerobic exercise three or four times per week, you can have great looking, muscular legs with these exercises.

Stand about two feet from one side of your bench (coffee table or whatever). Extend your right leg and rest your right calf across the top of the bench. Hold onto a chair or the top of the bench to support yourself or place your hands on your hips. Bend your right knee until your thigh is almost parallel to the floor. Return to the starting position, making certain you don't lock out the knee of your supporting leg. Do eight to 10 repetitions with one leg, switch and do the same number of reps with the other. Do at least three sets for each leg.

You can also perform squats at home using one of your children or your wife for the load. Have them climb on your back, or on your shoulders if you feel confident enough, and with your back straight and your head forward, slowly bend your knees and lower your butt until your thighs are about parallel with the floor. Hold for a two count, and then return to your starting position. Do eight to 12 repetitions for three to five sets, once a week.

You can also work your calves in the same way. With someone on your back, stand on the edge of the first step, provided you have any stairs in your home, that is. Hold the hand rail for support and balance and slowly raise yourself on the balls of your feet until you are fully extended. Then lower yourself until your heels are slightly below the step, hold for a two count, and then repeat. Eight to 12 repetitions and three sets once a week, combined with the above exercises I've described, and your legs will be shapely and muscular in a few short weeks.

Chest: Doing slow-count pushups using your dumbbells as handles is an excellent chest-builder.

Place your dumbbells on the floor, parallel to each other, about slightly more than shoulder-width apart. Lie face-down between the dumbbells and grasp the handles firmly with your legs straight behind you, toes on the floor, heels up. Tilt your chin towards your chest to align your neck with the rest of your spine, then straighten your arms and push your body upwards.

From this position, bend your elbows slightly and slowly descend until you are just hovering slightly above the floor, but not resting on it. Tighten your abdominal muscles while you do this so your lower back doesn't sag. If you can, do eight to 12 repetitions and as the weeks go by increase this number until you can do a set of 20. Do three sets each time you perform this exercise. Eventually, you can add load by having one of your children, or your wife lie face down on your back while you perform these - by then you'll have a huge chest, however.

For variation, try elevating your feet slightly until they are at as much as a 45-degree angle, which will add load to the exercise and will work the upper chest muscles a little more.

You can also perform dumbbell flys if you have a suitable bench. Lie face up on the bench and hold your dumbbells in each hand, shoulder-width apart directly above your head. Slowly lower each arm to the side while slight bending your elbows until the dumbbells are parallel to your chest, and then push them upward again until they reach the starting position. The exercise should feel somewhat like you are "hugging a barrel" if you are doing it correctly. Three sets of eight to 12 repetitions, combined with the slow count pushups and their variations, once a week will give you great-looking pecs.

Biceps: These are easy muscles to work, even if you are working out at home. They respond quickly too, because they are short compared to some of the larger muscles of your body. These exercises are bicep curls.

Grasp your dumbbells in each hand and stand upright with your feet shoulder-width apart. You may want to wear a kidney belt for addition back support while doing these curling exercises.

One curl variation is to stand with your elbows just slightly touching your sides and slowly curl one dumbbell at a time towards your shoulder. When it gets to this position, hold and slowly lower until it reaches its starting position. Do your arms alternately for one set, then simultaneously (if you're able - you may not be at first).

For variation, try hammer curls. Stand the same way, only instead of holding the weight with your palms toward you, hold them with your palms facing your sides. Curl the weight towards your shoulder only with your palm facing inward all the time. Again, when it reaches your shoulder, pause for a two count, then return to the starting position.

Another curl variation is the concentration curl. You can do this while sitting on your bench or on a chair or on the edge of the coffee table. With the dumbbell in your palm, rest your elbow up against the inside of your leg and place your opposite hand behind the elbow of the arm that is doing the exercise. Curl the weight towards your shoulder once again. It will be much harder to do the exercise this way, mostly because you are taking your back out of the mix so it concentrates all the effort on your bicep.

Again, do three sets of eight to 12 repetitions.

Back: An excellent exercise, known as the double arm pullover, will work most of the muscles in the upper-back region as well as some of those in the lower region too.

Lie face up on the bench with your feet hip-width apart on the floor. Hold a dumbbell in each hand (you might want to use less than 20 lbs in each hand to start with). With palms facing each other, arms extended upright, move the weights in an arc-like path (using your shoulder, not your elbows) until your elbows are about even with your eyes. Hold here until you feel a slight stretch or for a count of five, whichever comes first. Raise the weights to their starting position. Be sure not to arch your back during this movement. Do eight to 12 repetitions, and three sets.

For your trapezius muscles - the triangular ones in the upper, centre of your back which extend from the small region to the shoulders and neck - you can perform the upright rowing exercise using either one dumbbell held in both hands, or one dumbbell in each hand.

Stand upright with your feet about shoulder-width apart and your arms fully extended downward and your hands slightly in front. Lift your hands straight up towards your face, making certain they are parallel to your body the whole time. When they reach eye level, hold for a two count, and then slowly lower them again to the starting position. Again, do eight to 12 repetitions and three sets or more.

Finish your back workout with one of several good lower back exercises. You'll need a bench for both. Lie face down with your head even with one end of the bench and your legs hanging over the other end so they can touch the floor. Grasp the under part of the bench, or the sides, with both hands and hang on tightly. Flex your abdominal muscles tightly, and then raise your legs until they are parallel with the rest of your body and hold for a two count. Lower them to the starting position and repeat until you've done eight to 12 repetitions. Do three sets.

A variation of this is to lie with your legs on the bench and your upper body hanging over the end. You'll need someone to hang onto your legs or tie a long towel around the bench and put the backs of your ankles under the towel to anchor yourself.

Place your hands behind your head and slowly extend your lower back until your upper body is just parallel with your legs and hold for a two count. Again, do eight to 12 reps and three sets.

Triceps: For these longer, more graceful muscles in the backs of the arms, you can do several variations of the triceps extension exercise - either lying or sitting or standing - they all work the same way.

Lie face up on the bench, holding a dumbbell in each hand, palms facing inward, bend your knees and place your feet flat on the bench. Lift your arms so they are above your head and about shoulder-width apart. Keep your elbows straight, but relaxed and your wrists in line with your elbows. Keeping your upper arms stiff, bend your elbows and lower both weights at once until they are near your ears. Hold for a two count, and then extend the weights back to the starting position using only your tricep muscles.

Perform the same routine sitting but this time you can do one arm at a time while bracing your shoulder with the hand which isn't being used. The same goes for the standing version.

Another variation is one where you sit on the bench, keeping your back straight and hold one dumbbell in both hands, behind your head. Extend your hands until they are fully above your head using only the triceps to perform the exercise.

For any of these extension routines, do eight to 12 reps and three or more sets.

Tricep kick-backs are another excellent muscle for building size and strength in this area and for giving wonderful shape and sharp cuts to this muscle.

With one foot on the floor and the hand on the same side grasping the edge of the bench, place on knee on the weight bench and hold a dumbbell in the arm that is hanging free at your side. With the palm facing inward, keep your upper arm as still as possible and extend your wrist in a backward motion until it is parallel to the floor, using only the tricep muscle to complete the movement.

Do eight to 12 repetitions with one arm, then switch and do the same number of reps with the other arm. Do three sets or more with each arm to complete the exercise.

Shoulders: Among the wide range of should exercises you can perform with dumbbells at home are the shoulder salute and shoulder flys.

The salute exercise looks like a salute - hence the name. Stand with feet shoulder-width apart, grasping a dumbbell in each hand, palms facing inward. Keeping your arms straight and your elbows unlocked, raise your arms in front of you until they are slightly above shoulder height.

Flys work much the same way only you hold the weight at your sides and extend your arms straight out from the sides until they are parallel to the floor. This same exercise can be performed with the arms in front of the body and raised straight out, one arm at a time, or both at once, until they are parallel to the floor but straight out in front of your shoulders. Doing eight to 12 repetitions, one set of each variation, will give you a very complete shoulder workout.

As you get stronger and better at the exercises, perform as many as three sets for each exercise.

You can also perform the standard military press with dumbbells, which also works the shoulders very effectively. From either a sitting or standing position, grasp a weight in each palm with the hands parallel to the shoulders and slightly in front of your body. Raise each weight straight over your head for a two count, and then slowly lower it again. Alternate arms or do both at once - a few sets of both with give you a better workout.

Abdominals: Luckily there is a wide variety of good abdominal exercises that can be performed at home and among these are leg raises, the elbow-to-knee crossovers, crunches and reverse crunches.

122

To perform leg raises, lie face up on the floor with your hands by your sides, palms down and your legs together, toes pointing up. Raise your upper body until you are resting on your elbows in a semi-upright position. Then, raise both legs together until they arrive at an angle of about 45 degrees from the floor. Hold in that position for a two count, and then slowly lower them to a position about an inch or two off the floor so that your abdominal muscles must remain continually flexed. Repeat for eight to 12 repetitions and three full sets.

For the elbow-to-knee crossovers, again lie face up on the floor with your legs together, toes pointing upward and place your fingertips gently against each side of your neck. Don't be tempted to clasp your hands behind your neck because doing this will only injury your vertebrae as you struggle to lift your head to meet your knees. This isn't how the exercise works.

Instead, place the fingers of each hand on either side of the neck then move your right elbow upward and to the left to meet your left knee with will come up from the floor to meet it somewhere over your abdominal area.

Slowly lower both your elbow and your leg and repeat using the opposite elbow and knee this time. Keep your legs hovering an inch or two above the floor and your head suspended an inch or two above the floor as well to get the full benefit from this exercise.

You will want to do at least 15 repetitions on either side. Rest, then do another set until you've completed at least three sets. You should be able to feel this one by the time one set is completed.

The abdominal crunch is a similar setup, with the fingertips near either side of the neck. This time, cross your legs like you are going to sit cross-legged on the floor and raise your knees so they are perpendicular to the floor. Raise your head to your knees while at the same time bringing your knees forward to meet your forehead somewhere in the middle of your abs. A set of 20 reps and three sets should give your abs a good burn.

The reverse crunches are a bit tricky at first but once you get the hang of this exercise it really starts to carve out your mid-section.

Lie face up on the floor and put your hands behind your head. Grasp hold of a table leg or something that will anchor you and, with your feet together, raise your butt off the floor and your feet straight up in the air until you feel pressure on your abdominals. Hold for a two count and return to the starting position. Repeat this without stopping for 12 to 20 repetitions. Do three or more sets.

Finish your ab workout with side leg-raises, which will work your external and internal oblique muscles. Lie on your side with your top arm at your side and the palm of your underneath arm flat against the floor to help anchor yourself. Raise both legs, with your feet together until they are at a 45-degree angle from the floor. Pause for a two count, then return to the start position. Do 12-15 reps on both sides for each set and three or more sets.

This exercise for the obliques can also be performed with a dumbbell and is known as a side bend. Stand upright with your feet about shoulder-width apart. Hold a dumbbell in one had and place the palm of the other hand behind your head. As you stare straight ahead, bend to the side with the weight as far as you can, then return to the upright position. Do eight to 12 repetitions then switch the weight to the other hand and repeat on the other side. Do three sets on each side.

If you really want to bump up your home gym workouts a notch, try installing a chinning bar in a doorway or attach one to the rafters in the basement or even in the carport or garage if you have to. Nothing will tone and build your upper body like doing a variety of chin-ups - wide grip for the altissimo dorsi muscles of the back, narrow grip for lower back and trapezius muscles in the back, shoulder-width, reverse grip for the shoulders and triceps and negative chins for your biceps and forearms.

Incorporate one or more of these exercises into your routines for back, shoulders, triceps or biceps each week and be amazed at what a difference it will make in your upper-body shape. Just a few weeks at this and you will be more tapered, with wider shoulders, a narrower waist and a much broader back.

The best part about these exercise devices at home is that they cost so very little compared to a gym membership. On the other hand, the gym will offer more equipment for more body parts but as long as you stick with the program at home, you can look just as ripped as the guys in the gym look.

Home Gym Equipment

There are so many so-called complete home gym devices on the market these days that it's difficult to know where to begin. All I can say about this stuff is be sure you are getting something that is easy to use, won't take up too much space and will stand up to years and years of constant use. Remember, you aren't in this for the short term, but the long haul. It makes no sense to purchase cheap equipment on sale at the local department store if it won't last a year.

Well-made equipment by reputable manufacturers should come with a long warranty against failure. What's more it should perform a number of functions that will work every part of your body, including the legs. Stay away from circuit-training style devices that are a maze of cables and pullies. The more moving parts the equipment has, the more likely its chance of failure with repeated use. Home gyms are fine as long as they are working. If they are broken down you'll be forced to make the repairs yourself or find someone capable of coming into your home to do the repairs.

Some of the better equipment on the market is made by Nordicflex and Bowflex while aerobic equipment like stationary bikes and stairsteppers from Lifecycle and Lifestep are well made and do just what they were designed to do.

You can pay a little or a lot for this equipment so be sure you shop around and ask plenty of questions. Better yet, if you know somebody else who has good equipment they are happy with and which seems to be very durable, get what they've got.

Chapter 11
Attitude and Self-confidence

If you went without eating for an entire day, you would become hungry and your body would become weakened until you fed it again. Self-confidence also needs to be nourished on a daily basis in order to grow and get strong.

Accomplishment is a sure-fire method of feeding one's confidence so make a point of setting personal goals - either weight goals, food goals, fitness or discipline goals - and try to accomplish them in some small way every day. To do this, simply write down a list of things you wish to accomplish during that day, whether it be 20 minutes of aerobics, not eating any junk or fast food or whether it's getting to the gym on time and spending a pre-set amount of time working out. Then, go out and do these things and be proud of the accomplishments you have achieved in reaching each of these goals. Consider each accomplishment a "win" and get excited about it.

This may seem petty to a lot of people but it really isn't. In fact, it is essential as a first step towards nurturing self-confidence that may have been suffering from malnutrition for a long, long time.

Remember, these goals or promises are to yourself and it's only important to you that you honour each one. They are also the easiest to break since nobody but you is going to be hurt or suffer if they don't get accomplished. Be good to yourself, though, and honour these commitments to yourself.

Remember also to focus on progress, rather than perfection. The former is a concept that can be achieved on a daily basis and results in steady growth. The latter is just a wish or a dream - a fantasy, if you will - that cannot be attained and should never be part of your thought process.

Eventually, as time goes by and your body begins to respond to the new habits of good nutrition and daily exercise, you will become filled with a sense of self-worth and self-fulfillment that will boost your confidence to heights you likely never attained no matter how many deals you closed, how many cars you bought and how much money you might have made.

Once you trade pizza, beer and junk food for chicken breasts, egg whites, sweet potatoes, oatmeal and fish, once you trade soft drinks, processed food and bad water for essential oils, soy lecithin, apple cider vinegar and purified water, your life will be different, inside and out, and your confidence will soar.

Desire

Above all, you're going to need desire, the desire to make the necessary changes that will make you into a completely different kind of person - inside and out. Too often I hear men ask the question "how can I get in shape?" To this I reply, "Change your life!" Most of the time they either don't know what I'm talking about, or else they aren't prepared to make wholesale changes in their eating and living habits. Most guys are looking for the quick fix that is somehow going to magically undo decades of neglect and abuse. Well guess what? It's not going to happen that way.

The desire to become a new person, combined with nutritionally sound eating habits, a plan of action in the gym and some discipline will bring results quicker than you might expect. In fact, 10 to 12 weeks of steady work will transform anyone into a much leaner, healthier man. On the other hand, six months will do a much better job. What's more, once you've spent that kind of time working at the new you, you'll find that there is a willingness on your part to maintain a healthy well-being instead of slipping back into the sedentary, neglectful, lazy kind of existence.

Remember that nobody was born into this kind of lifestyle, it had to be learned, adopted and practised and the same goes for you. The "secret" to success is really no secret at all, nor is it exclusive. You can develop a belief in yourself and you can develop the confidence you need to move forward and overcome the obstacles that stand in our way.

Pretty soon you'll be steaming along, filled with confidence, knowing that no matter how bad the past has been, the future looks clean, bright and healthy. You won't have to stay in the comfort zone but will be filled with the confidence you need to take on bigger and bigger challenges and that you'll be constantly evolving - transforming - metamorphing into a better, healthier you.

Get Some Sleep

Plenty of rest and, in particular, plenty of good, sound sleep are essential if you hope to be successful in your desire to rebuild a new image from the inside out. If you are thinking that you can somehow build muscle mass in a state of almost constant sleep deprivation, it's going to be a nightmare!

Even if you are doing the right type of exercise and are following a good nutritional program, your body won't respond properly unless you are getting at least six hours of sleep each night - preferably seven or eight.

Scientists have found that not getting enough sleep causes significant unrest to many of the body's important biochemical systems, including the endocrine or hormonal system, and the immune system.

Stress can play a big role in sleep patterns and it's a fact that if you are a North American male, in mid-life, you likely have enough stress to sink a battleship. Luckily, vigorous exercise, combined with the right nutrition and daily supplements like essential fatty acids will go a long way towards easing some of the stress buildup. However, think about making some lifestyle changes that will get you out of those stressful environments a little more often. Add up the things that are important in your life and determine which of them you can safely do without. Do you need a bigger mortgage than you can carry? Do you need a second, third or even fourth vehicle, or do you need all those expensive toys in your driveway? Financial matters account for more stress than any other single source but it's one thing we have control over - or at least we should.

You can simplify your life by getting out of debt and to do this often only requires that we learn to live within our own budget and not well outside of it. Keeping up with the Joneses is still one of the prime motivating factors while staying fit and healthy seems to run a very distant second, if it's on the list at all. By now you've made up your mind to do something positive about your body image and your nutritional needs and this also means being good to yourself emotionally and mentally too.

All of which brings us around to the subject of sleep once more. Destressing your life, making it simpler and making it more clean and more fun are certain to have a profound affect on your sleeping life, not to mention everything else you do in bed - or used to do, for that matter. Learn to enjoy sleep once again, learn to welcome it at the end of the day.

Nevertheless, there can always be mitigating factors that prevent us from getting a good night's sleep. If you are drinking too much caffeine over the course of the day, and this is very easy to do since everyone's caffeine tolerance level is different, you might think about cutting back on the amount you are drinking. You might even switch to a decaffeinated brand of coffee, or order decaf latté and cappuccinos at the espresso bar you frequent on your way to and from the office.

Find ways to wind yourself down in the evenings as well as bed time approaches. Reading is better for unwinding and calming the mind and body than is watching television or videos, or talking business on a cell phone, for that matter. Conversation with your wife and/or children also works better as a calming factor in the evening, provided the conversation isn't forced or filled with dramatic conflict, that is.

Stay away from sleep-enhancing products or sleeping pills. These may knock you out but they don't provide your body with the kind of sleep you require for proper rest and recovery. One of the exceptions to this rule is melatonin which is a hormone secreted by the pineal gland in the brain during sleep and which is available as a supplement from most health food stores.

Melatonin is vital for the maintenance of normal body rhythms, especially the sleep-wake cycle and seems to play a vital role in many other body functions including the retarding of the aging process. It can be especially beneficial to men who travel a lot and who suffer from jet lag and other ailments that can disturb normal sleep patterns. Melatonin helps normalize the body's circadian rhythm, which regulates the sleep-wake cycles.

This hormone is produced by the body naturally but, like so many hormones, production decreases with age. As a result, many middle-aged men experience some form of sleep disruption or even sleep apnea and suffer a lot of related problems.

Unfortunately, melatonin isn't recognized by the food and drug agencies equally on both sides of the 49th parallel. It is available in Canada but you may have to ask your health food store employee on the sly to slip you some under the counter.

Anyway, the more sleep and rest you give your body, the calmer you can make yourself and the less stressed you can be, the better off everything is going to be in the short term and in the long run.

Chapter 12
Clothing And Gear

Any sport requires some preparation and some cost outlay and belonging to a gym is no exception. Aside from the membership fees, which vary dramatically from one location to another, you'll require some basic clothing and a minimum amount of standard equipment that will help speed you on the road to recovery and retribution.

If you look at your needs from the ground up, obviously footwear is the place to start. Most gyms have either in-house rules or health and safety regulations which prevent you from working out in bare feet, although if that's what you'd prefer and the gymnasium has no objection then feel free. However, it could get a little uncomfortable if you are pushing hard on a squat sled that has a knurled footboard.

The likely candidates for all-round gym and aerobic activity are the cross-trainer style sneaker, which comes in a wide variety of brand names and price tags. These shoes do provide an added measure of comfort and support for these activities, however, and are well worth the initial investment. If you are only wearing them in the gym, they will almost certainly last several years or longer before they need to be replaced.

A lot of weight trainers these days prefer something a little more heavy duty than the old cross-trainers and will opt for the ubiquitous construction boot, either in black or brown. These generally have steel shanks and steel toes which certainly offers a realistic measure of protection in an environment where a sizeable piece of cast-iron could potentially be dropped on your foot at any time.

This type of footwear also provides an added measure of support through the ankle area and this could conceivably come in handy if and when you begin doing leg squats with hundreds of pounds on your shoulders. They also have the most macho look to them - sort of a "no sissies allowed" type of thing, and this, too, can be a good thing, especially if you're just new to the place and want to look like you're going to fit in.

Inside whatever footwear you choose, make certain you wear a good pair of athletic socks. Not only do they keep your feet dry, they are also comfortable, especially if they are a cotton-lycra blend. Some prefer all wool socks but either way, make certain they are thick enough to help absorb some of the pounding and shock that is going to be sent their way over the course of your training sessions. A little foot powder sprinkled inside your footwear before each workout wouldn't hurt anything, either.

And one other thing, pick a neutral shade for your socks and after you've laced up your shoes, push the tops of the socks down so they have that "relaxed" look... it just looks better and less dopey, too!

Shorts are better than sweatpants, especially for weight training and spandex or spandex-lycra blend cycling-style shorts are preferable. If you object to the spandex look, or if it isn't too flattering to your figure in the early going, you can wear a second pair of cotton shorts over top of these. The reason is the spandex cycling shorts are cut and sewn differently than regular shorts, allowing more movement in the crotch area. They also flex and move with the motion of your lower body which is a great deal more comfortable over the long haul, believe me.

For a top, a two-stage or layered look also works best. The underlying layer should be a cotton singlet or muscle shirt, tucked into the spandex shorts. Over this, wear a fleece-lined sweatshirt that has been cut down at the neck and shoulders so it is sleeveless and without a neckline. Again, the layering will provide additional protection for your skin when you are working things like the hack-squat rack, or doing squats with a heavy Olympic bar balanced across your shoulders. The knurling on this bar can leave some pretty heavy red marks on unprotected skin, or skin that only has a single layer of cloth to protect it.

If you become too warm during your workout, you can always doff the outer piece of clothing and pull your muscle shirt out of your shorts to allow air to get up under your shirt and circulate around your mid-section.

One last thing concerning clothing... don't be tempted to wear a sweatband. Please. If you have to cover your head with anything, make it a bandana, tied "pirate-style." You'll draw far less attention as a possible geek.

A pair of weight-lifting gloves is another essential item of equipment. These are like cycling gloves in that they have no fingers and have a mesh back to them to allow air to circulate. Unlike cycling gloves, they generally have an extra-thick layer of leather in the palm area to accommodate heavy handling of knurled bars. They will save your hands from uncountable blisters and will save them from becoming overly calloused. There are some who prefer to work out without gloves, but there are also people who wear tweed suits without underwear. Get yourself a good pair from the gym pro shop or any local athletic supply shop.

Another useful item, and one which you should have, is a kidney belt. These are extra thick through the back so they give addition support to your lower back and kidney areas when you are doing leg squats or bicep curls. However, this item can certainly wait a few months until you build up to the heavier weights. A good one isn't cheap but it will come in handy.

You might also want to invest in a pair of wrist straps, which are nylon or cotton straps with a loop at one end that go over the wrist. The other end is wrapped around the dumbbells or barbells to give you extra grip. With these you can squeeze out a few extra reps even after you become tired and begin to lose your grip on the bars.

The last piece of necessary equipment, other than a gym bag in which to carry everything, is a good water bottle. Get one that holds a litre, or as close to a litre as possible so that you are able drink purified or distilled water throughout the course of your workout to prevent dehydration. Get in the habit of having a pull on your water bottle after every set, just in case you forget.

Just another word of caution; don't drink coffee or cola soft drinks or slush drinks from your local convenience store while you are warming up, working out or doing your aerobic activity.

The sugar and/or caffeine in these beverages do absolutely nothing for you. In fact, the reality is quite the contrary. The sugar you are ingesting at the time will be used as energy - some of it, at least - and the rest will be stored as fat, thereby having the complete opposite effect that you are trying to achieve.

If you've already been going to the gym faithfully, but making a habit of drinking these beverages before, during or afterwards, you now know why you aren't getting anyplace. You've got to give yourself every chance possible.

Chapter 13
Stress And Other Detriments

We all have stress in our lives whether it's the day-to-day stress of getting to work on time, dealing with bosses, dealing with clients, dealing with customers, partners, spouses or the guy in the car beside you. It can also be in the form of envy, jealousy, sympathy, empathy or any of the other responses that make up the emotional senses.

Stress has been widely blamed for making North Americans sick these days, but how we handle stress is more important than how much stress is in our lives - at least to a point.

Living in an urban environment is naturally more stressful than living in a rural or suburban environment. Some occupations are naturally more stressful than others, too. Believe it or not, making too much money can be just as stressful as making too little - more, in fact.

Stress alters the chemical responses of our brains, which systematically affects all our bodily functions too. It triggers the release of adrenaline - the fight or flight hormone secreted by our brains - which cause your neck, shoulder and abdominal muscles to tighten up and your breathing to become shallow, rapid and high in your chest. It is these reactions that are our bodies' responses to fear, anger, stress, sadness and physical pain.

A continuous amount of stress in your daily life will mean your breathing is almost always of the shallow type and this does not allow enough oxygen to reach the bloodstream and therefore not enough reaches all the areas of the body, including the brain and the muscles. This shallow breathing also accounts for fatigue, insomnia, anxiety, panic, muscle cramps and even intestinal gas, sometimes.

By learning to relax more and breathe deeper - both consciously and unconsciously - we can guard against the accumulative and negative effects stress will have on our bodies. Deep breathing strengthens vitality while shallow breathing depletes it. By breathing deeply and completely, the additional, fresh oxygen will help to counteract the stress and will help to calm your mind and spirit.

And believe me, oxygen is a vital component and a vital energy source. We can last without food for months, without water for days but without oxygen for only minutes.

This is one of the reasons why aerobic activity is so healthful because it allows us to get our focus off the stressful things in our minds while elevating the heart and respiratory action so that we are breathing deeply.

However, we have other ways of dealing with stress that are intrinsic. Studies have proven that those who have a sense of control over their lives, and who are optimistic, are able to keep their stress chemicals from reaching damaging levels when they are under pressure. Those who feel a sense of having no control over their lives, by contrast, succumb much more easily to stress and it's damaging affects.

Also, if you feel that what your are doing has value and importance, that you have a sense of purpose to your life and to your activities, then you'll deal with stress much easily and more effectively than someone who is pessimistic and anxious and out of control.

This entire process is what's known as coping. How you cope with stress determines how it will affect you. People who cope poorly have a decreased immune response because anxiety and depression suppress immune activity making them more prone to the negative health effects. Acute stress can lower the number of white blood cells in the immune system as well as the levels of interferon, a chemical that prevents viruses from reproducing.

So, how do we counteract all these negative effects? The best method is to immediately begin destressing your life - ridding yourself of as many of the pressures of day-to-day living as possible while at the same time elevating your sense of self-worth and self-importance. Easier said than done, right? It doesn't necessarily have to be this way if we all practice cleansing, balancing and preventative techniques to combat stress.

First of all, even if it seems hopeless - which it isn't, just remember that no matter what is wrong, no matter how big the problem may seem or how out of control the situation appears, the sun is still going to come up tomorrow morning.

Kidding around, joking, laughing and making light of serious situations is one of the best antidotes that can be recommended. Laughter and attitude can be very powerful cleansers and very powerful allies in the never-ending battle against the forces of evil (stress).

Laughter does indeed have therapeutic value. People have been able to recover from serious illnesses and snap out of serious moods of anxiety and depression simply through laughter.

Laughing causes positive changes in brain chemistry by releasing endorphins and it brings more oxygen into the body with the deeper inhalations. Laughter releases tension, anger, fear, guilt and anxiety. A good laughing session can completely change your attitude. Knowing this, you might even want to invest in some classic episodes of Seinfeld or Cheers, which you can sit down and watch in times of severe anxiety or intense stress. Or, if everything seems hopeless one afternoon, take a couple of hours off and head to the movie theatre to see a good comedy - or duck into a comedy cafe or improv or just walk up to a stranger on the street if you have to, and ask him to tell you a joke. Even if he doesn't, the look on his or her face alone might be enough to make you laugh.

You might also consider keeping comic reading material around your home and/or office, even if it's joke books in the bathroom or cartoon books in the drawers of your desk.

Even if you can't manage to laugh, at least try to smile more often. In fact, think consciously of smiling more often at home, at work, in your car or at the gym or where ever you may be at the moment. Smiling is the precursor to laughter and increases feelings of happiness.

I know, personally, how therapeutic laughter can be, even in the face of insurmountable sorrow and darkness. I often reiterate this story to people who have gone through a period of bereavement or who are dealing with the loss of a friend, family member or close relative.

My own brother was tragically killed one hot August evening in 1978, taking one last fatal ride in an automobile with five friends - partying, having a good time and being teenagers, like all of us have done at some time in our early years. They were all killed instantly when the car they were riding in left the road and hit a boulder on the shoulder at more than 100 miles per hour.

Every member of my family was devastated, but none more than I since my brother and I were as close as could possibly be. In the days that followed, my grief only grew and the vast hopelessness that filled my soul was not just overwhelming but it was so physically apparent that I could barely breath and felt I too was dying, only I really didn't care since my precious brother was already gone. In fact, I welcomed the thought of leaving this world and joining him again - wherever it was.

Finally one afternoon, in a state of total despair and darkness I was sitting on the steps in front of my house sobbing with grief and was completely overcome with such intense emotion that I wasn't even aware of the world going on around me.

When I looked up there was a young man standing in front of me. He and his brothers shared an apartment below mine and we had occasionally shared a moment or two together and had shared more than a few laughs. However, we hardly knew each other and were as different as two people could possibly be. He was younger, filled with macho and bravado and was the central figure of a gang of toughs that spent their days recklessly partying and making fun of other people's misfortune as a way of entertaining themselves.

He was the last person in the world I would have expected would be the one to save me from myself at that moment. Possibly he had come across me by accident that day, and somehow sensed the same thing . . . that here was a man drowning in a sea of emotional trauma, and that if anyone was to do anything about it, it would have to be him. I know now that it couldn't have been easy for someone so used to being careless with other people's feelings to suddenly be the saviour for someone who had no

138

feelings left, other than complete sorrow. But he was the one who calmly reached into that inky abyss and pulled me back out.

First he sat beside me and pulled me into his chest, wrapped his arms around me, and simply hugged me like I was his only friend in the world. After a little time he talked about his own father's death many years before, and how he had cried so much he didn't think he'd ever have tears left for anything for the rest of his life.

Then he just switched the conversation to something light - something that was going on in the street at that moment - and began making sarcastic remarks about the situation. In a few minutes he had digressed into complete random silliness.

In a little while after that I, too, was laughing along with him and by the time we parted company an hour or so after that, I was once again filled with living and with the spirit of life.

He became my best and most trusted friend. Somehow, when he stretched out of his own comfort zone to help someone he hardly knew, it changed him, too, insomuch as he knew he could never go back to being the callous, uncaring and sarcastic person he had been for most of his life to that point.

Some 20 years later, he was tragically killed as well. By then, he was the most talked-about, gifted, incredibly funny person and best friend to so many people and family members that his funeral filled the church, and spilled out onto the street in both directions.

And I had my opportunity at that time to thank him for his gift to me and at the same time had the opportunity to change the hearts and lives of all those people. I was chosen to give this man's eulogy and in doing so, I reiterated the story of my brother's death and how he had saved me. Then I told the funniest anecdotes I could recall about the man we were burying that day. In a little while, the tears and agonized faces in the church that day changed to smiles and laughter. His own remedy for a serious situation had come full circle.

Clearly, laughter can make all the difference in the world but so too can your attitude. I learned plenty about both from a man who walked on this earth for just 37 years and a brother who lived for only 16.

Destressing Yourself

Let's make a big effort now to get rid of some of the unnecessary stress in our daily lives - not that there is a necessary kind of stress we must live with, only that there can be a reasonable amount around without altering things too drastically. Besides, getting rid of some will help us deal and cope better with what stress is left over.

First of all, take a long vacation from your occupation at least once a year, or more often if you can. The rest of the year, take small vacations - a couple of extra days here and there, perhaps added to long weekends to make mini-vacations.

Don't always plan to get away when you take a vacation either, even though this can be therapeutic, it can also be just as stressful, planning and executing a detailed travel itinerary.

Staying put can be just as relaxing, if not more so. Hang around the house, enjoy reading the papers or a few good books and catch up on your Jeopardeze (watching Jeopardy) or whatever it is that you enjoy most about everyday life even when you have to work the next day. Don't wear your watch when you're on vacation but instead run your life according to how you feel at that particular moment. Really practice living in the moment, too by doing things spontaneously or entertaining yourself in any way you feel fit to indulge in at the time.

Go for walks in your neighbourhood, get out on your bike or on your inline skates or do a little downhill or cross-country skiing or take up snowboarding if you've never tried it.

Take up a hobby - besides weight lifting - and spend some time each day or several times a week indulging in that pastime.

Listen to music, because music can soothe your mind, body and spirit like nothing else can. Music can also instill a passion within your soul that no amount of money, no amount of material wealth and no amount of fame and fortune can take the place of. This kind of passion can extend your life by many years and can keep you thinking and feeling young every bit as much as exercise and nutrition. If you want visual evidence of this, rent the video entitled "The Buena Vista Social Club." In that film, produced and directed by Ry Cooder, a few dozen aging Cuban jazzmen are reunited after more than 40 years apart. When they get together again, it's like no time has passed - even though they are in their 70s, 80s and 90s by this time. They are still passionate about their music, their singing voices are as crystal clear as angels, and they still play their instruments like they just finished their last gig the night before. It's inspirational to see their passion for life and living manifested in their love for music and in their gift for entertaining.

More than anything else, it drives home the fact that embracing a passion for anything can lead to passionate longevity.

Another stress-inducing item in our lives is the automobile. Most North Americans own at least one, most more than one and fully half the households have two or more sitting in their driveways. This means dealing with traffic and all the problems associated with it - noise, anger, frustration, traffic jams, accidents, parking, parking tickets, traffic violations, maintenance, repairs and yadda, yadda. Most of this means plenty of money out of your pocket too in the form of car payments, lease payments, insurance costs, operating costs such as fuel, oil changes, new tires, repairs etc. There are also parking costs, the cost of fines the cost of bridge tolls, highway tolls and hidden costs in everything and anything to do with an automobile. And if you think all this doesn't add up to a heaping helping of stress, think again.

Personally, I don't drive anymore. I still enjoy driving, don't get me wrong; however, one day I realized all the above-mentioned things were driving me crazy and adding in a huge way to the day-to-day stress that was sucking the life out of me. Then I sold my car, bought a transit pass and my stress level dropped by about 40 per cent... overnight!

Now I enjoy riding the bus because it's a much more social atmosphere and less stressful way of getting to and from work each day. My kids ride free with me on the weekends and anyplace I could go in a car, I can get to in the bus just as easily, if not quicker in most cases.

Certainly it's a little less convenient and there are a few adjustments that must be made in your life, but in the big picture, it was a great move. What's more, I run into more and more people every day who have decided to do the same thing. We like to think we are helping out the environment too, by putting less fossil fuel emissions into the atmosphere. And boy, are we saving a bundle of money in the process! You simply wouldn't believe how much money you are spending on a car, or cars, until you no longer have them. The difference is almost unimaginable... enough to take several long all-expenses-paid vacations every year, plus pay all your transit costs and buy a new bicycle and inline blades as well.

And everything else in our lives is only stuff. Stuff accumulates like nothing else does. Even if we get rid of all our stuff today, within a year we'd have just as much stuff accumulated. With this in mind, detach yourself emotionally and spiritually from all your stuff because it is of no consequence to the quality and value of your life. Your life is now and how you choose to live it, and how much you enjoy it, and what you get out of life is in no way measured by how much stuff you have gathered by the time you die.

And don't live your life for your job or your career. These are only a means to an end and again they are no measure of your self-worth or your self-confidence. Some of the richest, most successful and most powerful men in North America have still committed suicide. At the same time, some of the richest, most powerful, and most successful men in America have also volunteered to fight in wars, and laid down their lives, for something that was only a concept in their minds; something that they valued more highly than all the material riches imaginable.

A professional hockey player by the name of Pat Lafontaine - a gifted star and one who was paid handsomely for his services, too - illustrated this concept once. He and a few fellow players - most notably tough-guy enforcer Rob Ray - volunteered their time and services to construct a special annex to the Memorial Coliseum in Buffalo, N.Y. so that invalid, wheel-chair-ridden and otherwise underprivileged and severely challenged individuals could have a place from which they could watch their National Hockey League team play. These players not only helped build the special area, but also paid for its construction out of their own pockets.

When asked about his selflessness, Lafontaine simply shrugged his shoulders and said that how many goals he scored, how many points he accumulated in a hockey season made no difference to anyone in the long run. However, if he could die one day just knowing that he was somehow able to make a difference, that he could feel good about his life in some way, would be more of a measure of his success as a human being than anything he could accomplish on the ice. He said it in a sincere manner and in watching him, and listening to him, I couldn't help but feel he meant every word he said. It was another inspirational moment in my own life.

How about yourself? Would you consider yourself to be everything you are now even if you had nothing in your pockets or would you feel naked without your money, or without your car, or without your possessions? Perhaps you might want to reassess your life if you aren't happy with the answer.

A Positive Attitude

Our bodies have miraculous powers to heal on their own, without the advent of medicines and prescription drugs, doctors and medical services. Sometimes our own negativity shuts down this healing capacity, however. A positive, hopeful attitude can be cleansing and detoxifying. You can help this process immensely by practicing positive affirmation and positive thinking on a daily basis.

For instance, encourage concentrating on "rights" rather than "wrongs" and look forward to new activities and hopes rather than dwelling on the past.

Give your body and mind positive messages to heal and work on increasing your self-esteem and increasing your confidence in your coping ability.

Try to remove the emotional blocks in your mind that prevent you from healing and from attaining a better, more positive self image. Forgive yourself for anything you feel you have done wrong in the past and forgive people - any people, whether they are friends, enemies, family members or strangers - for wrongs you feel they may have done you in the past.

Forgiveness is good for the soul but so is confession. Sometimes telling someone - anyone - about your problems will make you feel better and will make those problems seem less overwhelming. Getting these things out into the open, instead of keeping them locked in your mind, will transform them into concrete items rather than something that is only a concept. Once they are objects, out in the open, they can be attacked from more angles and either defeated or reduced to smaller problems with fewer consequences.

Talk to someone about what's bothering you. Talk to a friend, talk to your wife, talk to your parents, your children, your pastor, your boss, your co-worker, the person who operates the elevator, and the person who drives the bus or simply talk to a stranger. It works.

Sometimes, as in the case of a death of a family member or something equally traumatic, we need only to put our lives into the proper perspective - to get a little levity back into our lives. Think about what your life would be like right now if you suddenly lost someone near and dear to you - a wife, a child, a close friend or close relative. The currency of life is cheap and fragile. Don't take anyone for granted and be sure that other person knows how you feel about them before it's too late - for either of you.

And on the road to your spiritual healing, remember to indulge in random acts of kindness. Do something for someone simply because the opportunity exists to do it, not because it will improve your status or advance your station in life. Be kinder and gentler and keep your karmic tank topped up at all times, because one day the giant karmic wheel is going to turn around and come back your way. The universe is balanced in this way but only if you are balanced as well.

Chapter 14
Personal Appearance And Hygiene

Since your body image is going through a very dramatic change, it's time you also started to take control of other areas, too.

Cleanliness, good grooming, and taking care of your skin are things that a lot of men take for granted. Sometimes they will even rely on the advice of their wives, mothers, or girl friends for their personal care and maintenance. But, this is about taking control of your own body, your own mind, and your own spirit and these philosophies naturally extend as well to these areas. Chances are, you've never done anything for your skin in your life - or if you have, it was only to slap on a little after-shave lotion.

Your skin is an important and vital organ in your body and nothing else says that you are healthy, fit and vital than smooth, well-cared-for skin with nice texture, a soft, supple feel to it and, as much as possible, devoid of wrinkling and age spots.

Skin Care

Nothing makes a man look older than dry, wrinkled skin, devoid of life and having no shine or elasticity left. Skin performs necessary functions other than beauty. For instance, it helps regulate body temperature and retains body fluids. It is also the body's first line of immune defense against bacteria, viruses, fungi and foreign bodies.

Unfortunately, with age comes an inevitable slowing down of collagen formation. Collagen is a protein that is responsible for the resiliency or elasticity of the skin. This change is so gradual that most people - especially men - hardly notice it is happening until it is virtually too late to halt the process or do anything to remedy the damage that has already taken place.

At the same time, forces of gravity are working on our skin, pulling it southward and making it seem looser and somewhat flabbier. Less sebum is formed on the surface of the skin. This is protective oil secreted by the skin to hold in moisture and to form a protective coating. Cell generation also slows down which can leave skin looking drab and tired.

Meanwhile, the UVA and UVB rays from the sun - the ultraviolet light - damage skin cells, causing wrinkles, premature aging and, in the worst cases, melanoma or skin cancer. In fact, men are four times more likely to get skin cancer than are women, not necessarily because of their   different genetic makeup, but because they are generally exposed to sunlight more often and for greater periods of time - usually without any protection from the harmful rays, either.

To make matters worse, cigarette smoke - including second-hand smoke - causes serious damage to the skin. One night in a smoky bar can actually add years to your appearance simply because of the damage the smoke causes to your skin. It's always advisable to have a good, long shower when you arrive home from a night in a bar, just to scrub the smoke residue and toxins from the surface of your skin before going to bed.

On the positive side, proper nutrition, a healthy lifestyle, use of skin products and supplements as well as general care and attention can help skin maintain and even regain its youthful, vital appearance.

It may seem like a good idea and people may think it's a healthy look, but tanning is one of the worst things you can do to your skin and should be avoided - especially going to commercial tanning salons. Tanning is the body's response to injury and this is never a good thing, even under conditions of very gradual exposure. Tanning lights bombard the skin with UVB rays, the kind that cause the most skin damage and wrinkling.

Avoid going out in the sun during peak summer hours of 10 a.m. to 2 p.m. Wear sunscreen with sun protection factor (spf) of 8 to 15 minimum. A good sunscreen should protect the skin from both UVA and UVB rays and should be applied at least a half hour before going outdoors into the sun to allow it time to be absorbed into the skin.

Sunscreens are all chemical-based and I never recommend any kind of chemical use - whether topical, internal or otherwise.

However, "chemical-free" sunscreens use titanium dioxide that reflects UV rays by sitting on top of the skin but not getting absorbed. If you want total chemical-free sun protection, choose either UV-protective clothing, which is widely available and is as much as 100 percent SPF, or use zinc oxide cream. The latter is sold in all drug stores and most supermarkets, and is marketed mainly as a diaper rash prevention and cure. It is safe to use, blocks the sun's UV rays entirely, and is actually beneficial to the skin.

If you simply must have a tan, apply one of the bronzer lotions that will make you look like you've just come in from the outdoors on a summer day. They also contain chemical agents but are far less damaging to the skin than is the real sun.

A brief exposure to the sun in the early morning and later afternoon or early evening, is all that is necessary to help your body produce Vitamin A.

Once you come out of the sun, shower off all the sunscreen and immediately apply a generous layer of aloe Vera gel - preferably an organic type. Later, apply another generous layer of moisturizing cream but be certain it isn't a petroleum-based kind. Stay away too from so-called skin moisturizers, which contain bee's wax, alcohol and other ingredients that are actually not beneficial to the skin at all. Anything with a petroleum base and/or alcohol as ingredients will actually do the opposite of what they were designed to do. They will actually draw moisture out of your skin and make it drier and more wrinkled over time.

The best type of skin moisturizers will have natural ingredients derived from plant bases and herbs. Comfrey, chamomile, grapefruit seed extract and aromatic oils in a base of cold-pressed olive oil is what you are looking for. And don't assume simply because of the price, that a skin moisturizer is going to be a good one. In fact, some of the top designer brands available are some of the worst for the skin. My recommendation is the Oyama hand and body lotion made by Okanagan Naturals of Vernon, British Columbia. They aren't widely available but you can get them by phone (250-558-3939), or find them on the Internet and order online if you have to.

My own experience is that I have used these skin-care products for almost a decade and my skin is always envied and adored by women I meet. When I introduce them to these wonderful products they soon incorporate them into their own lives to the exclusion of all else. What's more, they are extremely inexpensive by comparison to almost anything else on the market today.

If you wear sunglasses, spend the money to get either prescription lenses or buy the expensive glass lens varieties. Cheap sunglasses often don't block out UV rays, are seldom polarized and usually diffuse the light in a manner that is more harmful than the rays, themselves.

If you live in a dry region, where the air is arid and the sun is intense during spring and summer, put moisturizing drops in your eyes occasionally during the day. If your eyeballs become dry and there is any friction, you can develop what's known as pinguequla. This is a condition whereby yellow fatty deposits build up in the corners of the eyes, resulting in red, itchy eyes that will eventually be very sensitive to light. If this conditions gets too bad, these deposits can potentially grow over the pupils and eventually must be removed surgically - a very painful process, believe me.

Wear a hat or cap as much as possible, not just if you are losing your hair and want to cover up or reduce the affect of wind blowing the arrangement out of order. A hat shields your scalp from cancer-causing rays of the sun.

A good idea also is to try finding a hair gel or cream that incorporates an SPF 15 sunblock as well. If you can't find one, put a dab - about the size of a dime - of zinc oxide cream in your palm and rub it thoroughly through your hair and massage it into your scalp. This will prevent sunburn of the scalp and will prevent your hair from drying to the consistency of straw in the summer sun.

Cleanliness

Everyone had a mother who used to preach the philosophy that cleanliness was next to Godliness, just before she would root out your ears with a soapy washcloth. It turns out that mothers knew what they were talking about - mostly, anyway. Too bad her words didn't get through to your father often enough, though. It seems when we were younger, our fathers somehow smelled a little less than fresh every day and it was because there was too little onus placed on good, old-fashioned cleanliness - as in taking a shower or a bath every day, sometimes more often in summer or if there were some kind of strenuous activity taking place like mowing the lawn or working on the house.

It was the kind of thing that created a stigma about men and their hygiene and these days there is often little to dissuade people from thinking otherwise about middle-age men. It only takes a few to give us all a bad name.

The truth of the matter is that viruses, fungi, bacteria, protozoa, disease and all sorts of infections and communicable nastiness are easily passed from person to person these days because we often share equipment in an office environment with one another. A computer mouse, a telephone, door handles, elevator buttons and so on and so on. No wonder North Americans are becoming chronically ill.

The easiest and simplest way to maintain your good health is to make sure your hands are clean since most of these viruses, bacteria and the like are carried to the infectable regions of the head by the hands - the eyes, the mouth, the nose and ears. Consciously washing your hands every hour or 45 minutes at the office will help to break this chain of infection from spreading. When leaving the bathroom, use a piece of paper towel to pull open the door handle, too.

Of course these same hands then put food in your mouth at coffee time, lunchtime and sometimes throughout the day if you snack at your desk or on the job as people often do.

The same goes when you are in the gym. Gymnasiums, regardless of how clean they are kept, are breeding grounds for bacteria - in common shower drains, sinks, toilets, and most especially on the equipment itself since it is used communally. All those hands grabbing barbells, dumbbells and handles add up to a lot of germs and bacteria. As soon as you've finished your workout, be sure you shower thoroughly or, if you prefer to shower at home, first wash your hands with warm water and soap before you leave the gym. Don't pick up anything and place it in your mouth before you have at least done this much.

What's more, the shower floor in a gym is a likely place to find the dermatophyte fungus, which causes athlete's foot. Be sure to wear rubber slip-on sandals (flip-flops) in the shower.

If you use the toilet at work, in the gym, at the office, or in your workplace, be aware that the flush handle, faucets and doorknobs can be tainted with fecal bacteria, including such delights as shigella, E. Coli, and salmonella. If you somehow introduce these to your mouth later, there's a chance they could cause diarrhea.

The same goes if you are shaking hands with people a number of times each day. Shaking the hand of someone who has a cold virus, then rubbing your nose up to an hour later and you've likely just caught what he had

Most gyms these days insist you wipe down any equipment after you've been using it and they even supply paper towels and disinfectant in spray bottles for just such purposes. However, even though a gym bench or aerobic cycle may be covered in sweat, it isn't necessarily dangerous because the salt in sweat inhibits the growth of most bacteria. Nevertheless, wipe it off for the next guy because it's only polite.

Avoid using commercial brands of hand soap on your skin. In fact, stop using them altogether except for washing your hands. These are too harsh and contain astringents that strip all the oils and sebum from the skin while penetrating to leave a residue.

Instead, use a shower gel that contains plant and herbal-based ingredients and natural fragrances. Again, Okanagan Naturals markets one of the best in the world and it contains purified aqueous extracts of aloe Vera, glycerine, orange oil, peppermint oil, grapefruit seed extract and other natural ingredients which work to condition and moisturize, soften, refresh and rejuvenate the skin while controlling bacteria and micro organism growth. There are others on the market that may contain many of the same ingredients, so shop around until you find a good one.

When you shower, place this gel on a shower puff, which is an item that looks like a bunch of fine mosquito or fish netting bunched together. These work to gently exfoliate the dry, dead skin cells from the surface of your skin while you clean yourself.

As for deodorant, get rid of any commercial varieties you may currently be using. As we mentioned previously, these contain harmful chemicals and toxic metal ingredients that can actually damage your health. Switch to a deodorant crystal - available in health food stores - or a deodorant crystal spray which comes in a non-aerosol spray bottle, and usually contains aloe Vera in addition to the crystal stone. These products are fragrance-free, hypo-allergenic, and non-staining without harmful chemicals, propellants or perfumes.

As an added bonus, they can also be used on the feet to counter foot odours.

Help for Hair Loss

If you are like half the men in North America who are middle-aged, you are no doubt suffering from some degree of hair loss or, at the very least, some hair thinning. There are so many cosmetic techniques springing up to re-seed thinning patches on a man's head that it must now be the number one cosmetic surgery procedure on the globe.

If you have had this procedure done, hopefully it was performed by a reputable doctor and an established clinic. If not, you could spend more of your life wishing you'd never bothered, than you ever did wishing you had a full head of hair once again.

On the other hand, if you are happy with what you have, or if you'd at the very least like to stop losing any more of what you've got, there is plenty of hope - especially if you've already begun following the nutritional secrets contained herein.

Nutrition, and more especially, getting the right balance of trace minerals in your daily diet, will make all the difference in the world to the quality, quantity and texture of your hair, not to mention the health of your mane.

Unfortunately, most men don't associate either good nutrition or good grooming practices with their hair loss. But then, most men don't associate good nutrition with the general condition of their bodies, either.

Trace minerals like silica, zinc, copper, iodine, and others will go a long way towards strengthening what hair remains on your head and occasionally - and don't get your hopes too high at this point - the process can even reverse itself, unless you are suffering from male-pattern baldness from which there is supposedly no cure. Of course at one time they said the same thing about many conditions and ailments that plagued mankind.

Luckily, more money is spent on research into regrowing hair on men's heads, than is spent collectively on all the cancer research currently going on everywhere on earth combined. Isn't it comforting to know that you may die, but you'll at least go with the dignity of knowing your hair will be intact on your head... comforting, wouldn't you agree?

Nevertheless, the best they've come up with at this point are chemical-based items like minoxidol - which is marketed as either a topical product or an oral medication. Neither is worth the money anyone is paying for them, in terms of what they'll do for the hair on your head. If, on the other hand, you want to look more like the wolfman than you do Brad Pitt (hairless chest and all, I mean), then by all means invest in either of these two products.

Everywhere you look there is an endless array of snake oils and so-called miracle hair restoration formulas but virtually all of them are designed to remove your money from your pocket rather than regrow any hair on your head. Like so many other enterprising individuals, they've found that there's serious money to be made taking advantage of the baby boomer generation's reluctance to grow old.

If you are willing to admit they are a waste of time and money, then there are things that can work in your favour and which I happen to know work to a certain degree - first hand, of course.

First, there is a silica gel available as a vitamin supplement. It comes in liquid form and is sold in health food stores and vitamin centres. Not only is it nourishing for the scalp and the hair shaft itself, but it adds an incredible amount of volume to your hair almost the instant it is rubbed in. In fact, it can give your hair twice the volume it had before you put it in. It's best to put it in when the hair is dry and it quickly dries itself so there is no wet look and no greasy mess whatsoever.

You can also take a teaspoon every other day as a vitamin supplement and ingesting silica is just as good for hair growth from the inside. It's worth its weight in gold, regardless of how you decide to use it.

Another product, which works surprisingly well, is an herbal formula marketed through health magazines, and also available exclusively through General Nutrition Centre stores throughout North America (GNC). It's marketed in tablet form called Shen Min and although it is available through certain retailers, mainly in the Eastern United States, it is widely available online or through toll-free ordering procedures. Although the exact formula is less than important, the herbs are vaso-dilators that seem to work mainly in the crown area of the head - right where you'd want just such a product to work. The bottle claims at least three months of three tablets daily is necessary before any results are seen, but almost anyone who has tried the formula reports thicker, fuller hair within a few weeks.

So far, users I know, including myself, have been overwhelmingly satisfied with the results they've obtained. It's unknown if it works for everyone, but it seems the less hair you've lost, the better and quicker are the results.

Some scientific studies have concluded that too much salt in one's diet can result in hair loss. These scientists also conducted tests which proved somewhat inconclusively, that a reduction in salt in the diet, as well as removal of salt from the tissue, corrected many hair loss problems. With that in mind, be certain you shower and wash all salt residue out of your hair and off your scalp following a workout or aerobic session.

Getting rid of emotional strain and stress, combined with nutritional supplements like essential oils, trace minerals and a nutritionally complete diet each day will go a long way towards making your hair - however thin and/or dull, dry and listless it once was - thicker, more lustrous and healthy-looking. If you've been following this plan all the while you've been reading this book, in fact, there should already be a noticeable difference in your hair, regardless of how little, or even how much of it you had to being with.

Still, if you'd care to give it every chance possible, you might also try taking cayenne pepper as a daily supplement. Take several capsules several times a day, with meals - never on an empty stomach. The cayenne seems to work as a powerful vasodilator and you'll know this by the warm feeling it creates in your body. Be warned, however, that bowel movements can be a little uncomfortable until you get used to the effects of the pepper on your system.

Apple cider vinegar, used as a topical solution, can also stimulate hair growth when it is applied to the surface of the scalp, then massaged in until a warm, tingling sensation is felt. This wonderful compound can actually aid hair growth because it draws blood to the area it has been applied to which, in the case of hair growth, is exactly the benefit you wish to achieve.

This process is best done just prior to retiring for the night since it will leave your head smelling just a little peculiar. While it will be fine if you are at home alone, or in the company of family members, it's doubtful if this aroma will go over too well in an office environment or any other confined area. Upon awakening, you can simply shampoo your hair when you shower which will easily get rid of the smell. You can also rub the vinegar into your scalp a half hour or so before you shower which will also benefit your scalp and your hair growth though the longer you leave it in the better will be the effect.

Old-fashioned and proven methods of stimulating hair growth also include massaging the scalp with the fingertips and giving it a good, thorough brushing several times each day.

Aloe Vera gel has also been known to stimulate new hair growth and to retard hair loss. Again, Aloe Vera gel is readily available in an array of sizes from health food stores and is relatively inexpensive, even for the organically grown varieties.

Kelp, as a supplement, can supply much-needed iodine to your daily diet, which, in turn, helps stimulate abundant hair growth.

Most of all, getting as much stress out of your life as possible is the best antidote to hair loss. Stress is the major cause of early hair loss and rapid hair loss in later years. It seems the older we get, the more stress we have in our lives until, at middle age, we are dealing with stress levels far and above those we had to deal with as young men.

If you think stress is unimportant in the process of hair loss, go downtown sometime and take a look at the homeless drunks that wander the streets and inhabit the decaying urban areas. If you find one that doesn't have a great head of hair, I'd be very surprised. These guys, most of whom have fallen through the cracks in society because of their drinking problems, have almost all arrived at a station in life where they are able to concentrate on just one thing - getting something to drink each day. All the other stressful components of their lives have been virtually removed from their minds. The result is they suffer little or no hair loss in spite of the fact that they have very bad diets and are nutritionally nowhere.

Shampoos and Hair Gels

When we were discussing effects of the sun on the body earlier, it was also mentioned that rubbing zinc oxide cream into your hair was a good idea to prevent sun damage. However, the zinc is also absorbed into the scalp and this is beneficial to your hair as well. It can add a great deal of volume to your hair as well and I like to use it as a sort of super hair gel. It seems a tad greasy at first, but after a few hours it seems to dry fine with no matting or sticking. This might not be for everyone, however.

Another ideal hair gel is the hand and body lotion mentioned earlier as well. With its list of wonderful natural ingredients, it seems to bring life to anyone's hair. I've even talked women into using it as a gel and, though reluctant at first, they've been amazed at the wonderful results they've obtained with its use. This lotion also leaves your hair dry in a brief while so don't be alarmed if it seems a little greasy at first - it's only temporary, if at all.

Silica gel is also a wonderful compound that is highly recommended. However, all commercial hair gels contain chemicals as well as fragrances and other toxic ingredients that, when used over a long period of time, will accumulate on the shaft of the hairs making your hair dull. Remember also that anything you apply topically to any part of your body will eventually be absorbed to some degree. What this new philosophy is all about is getting rid of toxic chemicals and detoxifying your body, not adding new ones to the list. Therefore, simply avoid using these commercial hair gels, thickeners (unless they contain natural ingredients) and all other compounds that will be detrimental to the health and well-being of your hair and yourself.

This goes as well for commercial shampoos. Regardless of what they claim in their advertisements regarding their ingredients, virtually all these shampoos contain chemical compounds and toxic agents that are neither good for your hair nor good for your health in general.

Again, health food stores carry a wide variety of shampoos, conditioners, gels and other hair ointments, creams and lotions which contain natural ingredients and are made without commercial detergents which strip the hair and scalp of all essential oils and humectants.

Chapter 15
Get Into Your Kitchen

Your grocery shopping list is going to be a little different from now on and you may have to do a little searching to find the right kinds of food and supplements you're going to need on a daily basis for your new lifestyle and the maintenance of your new body.

Fruit and vegetables: Whenever and wherever possible, switch your fresh fruits and vegetables for those that are organically grown. There are more nutrients in organic produce and fewer toxins, herbicides, fungicides, pesticides and so on to be ingested. Eating fruit and vegetables purchased from the produce sections of huge supermarket chains will only help to continue the process of toxification, which has probably been ongoing for most of your adult life already. You don't want to start adding to the problem, you want to begin the solution and the best way to do this is to simply choose organic. You'll notice the difference quickly, believe me.

However, if organic fruit and vegetables are difficult to find, out of season in your part of the country or for reasons beyond your control, simply can't be found, take some precautions before eating the non-organic variety. At the very least, wash them thoroughly with fresh, purified water - preferably distilled. The best solution is to soak them in a bath of water and one of the many fine products available now for washing produce. These were once available only at health food stores - and still are. However, due to the increasing demand, some of the bigger corporations, like Proctor & Gamble, for instance, have now begun marketing a fruit and vegetable wash that is made of natural ingredients and is biodegradable and harmless for human consumption. These are very effective at dissolving toxic chemicals and/or chemical fertilizers that are on the skins of this produce. They also remove up to 95 per cent of the wax that coats many fruits and some vegetables that are sold in supermarkets.

Many of the larger grocery chains now feature organic produce, but if they don't, insist they begin bringing it in for you... this might work, especially if they've already had previous requests. This kind of produce is readily available at health food stores and almost every community in North America has at least one of these nowadays.

Always have fresh carrots and fresh spinach on hand for juicing, for putting into recipes, or as healthy raw snacks. Spinach was once only a seasonal vegetable but now is available year-round in pre-packaged plastic bags, which come from California and Mexico in winter. Just be certain this type is organically grown, because countries like Mexico have a different set of agricultural rules to follow where fertilizers, and chemical inhibitors are concerned. When it is in season in your area, take advantage. The same goes for any fruits and vegetables native to your area when they are in season.

You'll also need to have sweet potatoes or yams around, regular potatoes, bell peppers - all colours, including red, green, yellow, brown and any others they may now have on the market. String beans, snow peas, bok choy, broccoli, cauliflower, Brussels sprouts, asparagus spears, beats and onions - white, red and green varieties - are all staple vegetable items you'll want to have on hand in the produce drawers of your refrigerator. And while you're at it, don't forget to have a plentiful supply of organic, ripe tomatoes on hand as you'll want to include these in your daily diet for the benefit they will have on your urinary tract and prostate gland.

Remember, if you have any of these vegetables for any length of time and they begin to dehydrate, bruise or begin to deteriorate, simply put them through your juicer and enjoy the results. In this way you can save money by not throwing out veggies and fruit you might otherwise be inclined to toss.

Fruits to have on hand include apples, pears, strawberries, raspberries, apricots, peaches, mangos, papaya, kiwi, blueberries, bilberries, cranberries and bananas. All of these can be eaten raw, some of them can go into your blender drinks and smoothies to add important enzymes and flavenoids, and some of them can be used in cooking and juicing. Apples, for instance, are great to add to your juiced carrot and spinach concoctions to add flavour and to sweeten it up a bit.

Melons are another important source of enzymes, nutrients and, especially, organic water. There is an abundant variety available throughout the year but, as always, make your preference organic. Watermelon, canteloupe, honeydew, casaba, muskmelon and a number of cross-bred varieties - like honeyloupe (cantaloupe and honeydew cross) - are also excellent and delicious.

Again, these can be eaten as snacks and are a good idea to eat as a water-replacement after your aerobics or gym workout because their organic water content is high and their flesh can be easily digested and assimilated into the cells quickly.

They, too, can be put through a juice machine to add these important nutrients, enzymes and water to your carrot juice. When you put them through a juicer, leave the rind on as well since there are important trace minerals stored here but which are usually discarded when eaten.

Salad greens: The idea of making a salad is not only foreign to a lot of men, but the idea of actually eating one is often just as foreign a concept. Luckily, there are pre-packaged salads these days that take all the guess work out of chopping, shredding and ripping apart salad greens in order to piece one of these things together.

Not that this can't be accomplished and even enjoyed. If you want you can purchase organically grown heads of romaine and fancy leaf lettuce, spinach and a host of other greens as well as a variety of coloured salad veggies and make your own. If you want to skip all this fuss, try purchasing organic salad greens in bulk from the organic produce section of your supermarket or purchase these from your local health food store.

They also come pre-bagged from such reputable organic producers as Natural Selection Foods out of San Juan Bautista, California (try their website at www.ebfarm.com for the nearest location where this mix is available). These wonderful pre-mixed salads include red and green romaine, red and green oak leaf, lollo (ros, tango), frisee, radicchio, mizuna, arugula, baby red chard and baby spinach. Other brands may contain any mix of these and a number of other greens mixed in. The result is a highly nutrition, delicious salad blend. All you need to do is open the bag, take out a handful and put it on a plate or in a bowl and add a tablespoon or two of the flax seed-apple cider vinegar dressing (see recipe at the end of this chapter), and you're in business. It is quick, easy, and nutritious.

Whole grains, legumes, nuts and seeds: Staples to have on hand include organic long grain, brown rice or organic brown Basmati rice. Purchase whole wheat and natural pastas made with organic ingredients whenever possible. You can also find organic, raw nuts and seeds in bulk food stores and health food stores and you're going to need a constant supply of these as well so stock up. You'll need to have on hand organic, raw sunflower, pumpkin and sesame seeds as well as organic, raw almonds, walnuts, cashews, Brazil nuts and hazel nuts. You don't have to have them all at the same time, however. Have one or two varieties on hand at all times, though, for snacking and adding to recipes. Nuts and seeds can be stored in airtight glass containers with rubber sealing rings around the lids.

You may also want to have a generous supply of dried fruits on hand since these provide all the nutrients and enzymes found in the fresh versions, but with much less of the water. On the other hand, they generally have an increased fibre content once they are dried. Dried fruits such as pineapple rings and papaya spears will benefit digestion greatly with their enzymes while dried fruits like prunes (dried plums), apricots, peaches, pears and apples have a high fibre and fruit pectin content in addition to their valuable vitamins, minerals and enzymes.

Milk, cheese and yoghurt: I don't recommend drinking milk for anyone. In fact, I'm a strong advocate for not drinking cow's milk at all, since it tends to create more health problems than it solves. Among other things, it can create a lot of mucous in the linings of the throat. For another, most people are either lactose intolerant - meaning they can't digest the sugars in the milk - or else they have an allergy to milk and milk products. Often people aren't even aware they have this allergy but they may break out in hives, get red marks or dark circles under their eyes, have trouble sleeping or a suffer from a host of other difficulties related to food allergies.

Nevertheless, if you have to drink milk or use it on cereals or cook with it or bake with it, there are a number of alternatives that might work for you.

You could try either a lactose-reduced variety, in which an enzyme has been added to help pre-digest the lactose, or another type in which live bacteria culture like acidophilus has been added. This can mix with the good bacteria in your intestinal tract to help digest more of the lactose, thereby relieving you of the problems associated with lactose intolerance.

Milk alternatives like soy milk and/or nut milks also are highly recommended. Soy Milk has come a long way in recent years, and is almost as readily available as cow's milk in most dairy cases at the supermarkets. These now come in various flavours, but the plain will do, since the flavoured types have sugars and artificial flavouring added which you don't need, especially at a time when you are trying to rid your body of these toxins which have been accumulating for decades anyway.

Nut milks aren't readily available but can be produced at home in a blender. Simply place a cup of raw nuts in a blender - any type, except peanuts - and add a cup or more of fresh, purified water. Blend at high speed for a long time - as much as three or four minutes, until the liquid in smooth and devoid of grit or lumps. If you aren't certain, stop the blender, place the liquid between your thumb and forefinger and rub them together. If it feels gritty, blend it some more until it is smooth.

Nut milks make excellent substitutes for cow's milk or buttermilk called for in baking recipes such as muffins, so experiment making and using it if you need to really break away from the milk thing.

Yoghurt is a very nutritious and delicious milk product and because of the live cultures that ferment the yoghurt, the lactose is reduced and converted to a more easily digestible form. However, flavoured yoghurts are high in sugar content and most brands have too many additives to make the ingredients homogenous and stable for a long shelf life.

Therefore, the only kind recommended is plain yoghurt, made from organic milk. You can add your own fruit to the mixture, if you absolutely need something sweet. It can also be added to blender drinks to give them a little more body and to introduce friendly bacteria to your intestinal tract on a regular basis. If you are completely non-dairy at this point or are completely lactose intolerant, there are also excellent yoghurts made from alternative milk sources such as goat's milk and sheep's milk, both of which are safer for human consumption than is cow's milk and much easier to digest as well.

Water: This is the most important ingredient for your daily life, and it's of the utmost importance that you pay attention to the quality and quantity of water you are drinking. If you aren't currently drinking purified or distilled water on a regular basis, you must do this immediately. Don't leave your health to chance by consuming tap water to which your municipality has added every chemical under the sun to kill bacteria and beef up the quality.

The easiest solution is to have a water filtration system installed in your home. These products are plumbed into your drinking water lines and the purified water - which has gone through a process known as reverse osmosis - comes out of a separate tap that is then installed over your sink. In this way you can use it as drinking water and for cooking too, since the chemicals in tap water can permeate the vegetables, rice, pasta and potatoes that you are cooking.

If you can't install a water filter in your home, have purified water delivered on a weekly basis to your house or apartment. There are plenty of companies out there that are happy to provide this service nowadays, and the cost is not too great, as long as you don't rent the refrigerating device they will want you to have. All you need is a handy little plastic pump device that fits on the end of the five-gallon containers in which the water is delivered. You can purchase one of these for 30 or 40 dollars, and can use it for years.

Health food stores and most super market chains now offer bulk purified water as well as bottled water in almost every size imaginable. The bulk water is the most cost-effective since you can refill your own five-gallon jugs for as little as three dollars or less. It's a lot less convenient than having someone deliver your water, but if it were "convenient" to take good care of your health, it wouldn't be such a huge problem.

On the other hand, if your source of water is ground water, lake water or well water, chances are it is much cleaner and safer than city tap water. However, I suggest you have an analysis done and if it shows even minute levels of heavy metals and trace minerals you don't want in your body, switch to something else, at least for consumption.

The toxicity of water can be ingested in more ways than simply drinking it. Showering in toxic water and washing your clothing can also leave the same chemicals on your skin, which can then be absorbed. I have known people who eventually traced the source of their health problems to this fact. Changing this can be a huge expense, however. One person went to the trouble of installing a commercial-sized water distilling unit in his basement so he and his family could cook, clean, shower and wash their clothing in pure water.

Again, you can change your life right to the molecular level if you have a mind to or if you have motivation. On the other hand, a few subtle changes, like simply drinking purified water, will make a huge difference in most people's health and well-being.

Meat, fish, poultry and meat substitutes: Stop shopping for beef and red meat byproducts such as hamburger and the ground types of meats. These are higher in fat content, and are generally made from cuts of meat that have been left lying around for some time, or which may have been swept off the butcher's floor.

If you have to have red meat, make it the exception rather than the rule, and choose the leanest cuts you can find. Before cooking, trim off all excess fat.

Choose boneless, skinless chicken breasts - preferably those raised naturally without hormone injections or antibiotics, if possible. If not, get ones that advertise they are water-free.

Also purchase fresh fish and seafood and eat these once or twice weekly for their protein content and also for their iodine and trace elements.

Stop eating processed meats such as bacon, ham, hot dogs, sausages, kolbasa, etc. because they all have a high-fat content, contain too many preservatives and nitrites, and are bad for your health in general. Say good-bye to the days when you might have chowed down on two or three hot dogs and a couple of sodas or beers at the sports games. In your new life you need wholesome, nutritious food and not old habits that created the problems in the first place.

Eggs are another staple of your diet, especially the egg whites. However, always seek out the free range eggs or eggs from chickens which have been raised on an organic mash. These days, most supermarket chains carry a wide variety of eggs, but this is a poor source, since even the ones from chickens raised on organic mash employ caged birds to do their laying, resulting in a product from a highly stressed critter. Still, if you haven't got a health food store handy, a farmer's market or an egg farm within reach, you can opt for the very best they may have to offer in the supermarkets.

If you are vegetarian, tofu is one of the best alternatives to meat, since it is high in good quality protein. It comes in either soft, medium or firm, and you can choose whichever style you need for whatever you are putting it into.

There are also plenty of excellent vegetarian meatless patties on the market now, some of which have the flavour and texture of meat, and others which can actually be placed on a barbecue.

Cheese also has vegetarian alternatives. Almost every type of cheese available, from Parmesan to feta can be manufactured from soy bean curd now and most of the health food stores and even a good number of super market chains are carrying these cheese alternatives.

Herbs and seasonings: If you are at all adventurous, attempt to keep a small garden of fresh herbs growing on your window sill or on your patio in which you cultivate herbs like dill, basil (any of the dozen or more varieties), parsley, chives, green onions etc. If you don't want to start growing these you can always find them already potted in greenhouses and at farmer's markets and it's nice to have really fresh herbs growing around the house for putting in recipes, salads and sandwiches.

However, you'll also want to have a good supply of garlic on hand and these come in a variety of size, shape and bouquet and there are plenty of places that sell organic so that's what you'll want to buy. They also have something called whole clove garlic now which comes in the form of small bulbs that don't need to have the individual cloves broken off and shelled, You just shell the whole clove and use it as is.

Fresh, organically grown ginger is also available easily these days and you should have some of this on hand for your juicer, for making teas and for adding to recipes from time to time.

Where spices are concerned, I recommend a wonderful product called Spike, which I've mentioned many times during the course of this book. It is a mixture of sea salt and 30 or 40 herbs and spices to make one delightful additive that will enhance the flavour of just about anything but is especially tasty on meat, fish, eggs, vegetables and a lot of other foods. You can purchase this in bulk or by the shaker bottle. I suggest you buy one bottle and a box of the bulk, so that you can keep refilling the bottle when it's empty - which is going to be often.

Other suitable all-in-one spices include Mrs. Dash and a number of similar products.

There is one more item that is a must in every refrigerator and this is salsa. Salsa can be made at home or purchased just about anywhere, from convenience stores to supermarkets to health food stores.

Salsa is filled with wonderful ingredients like tomatoes, red and green peppers and jalapenos, chilis, onions, garlic and cilantro. It makes a wonderful accompaniment to any starch, especially brown rice, potatoes and sweet potatoes. What's more, the combination of ingredients in salsa makes it an ideal food for raising metabolic rates and burning fat and calories - the hotter, the better.

Supplements: You're going to need a good supply of whey protein powder, or a good soy protein isolate powder, since you will likely be ingesting two or more blender drinks each day as a supplement to your regular diet. There are so many on the market now that finding a good one isn't as difficult as finding a good one that is also cost-effective.

However, a good protein powder shouldn't have a lot of carbohydrates mixed in. In fact, some of the better brands on the market - PVL, by Ultimate Nutrition and Natural Factors, for example - contain only two grams of carbohydrate per 28-gram serving. This also includes 22 grams of protein, 1.5 grams of fat and only 110 calories per serving. If you purchase in large volume - five pounds or more at a time, the cost is about 75 cents per serving or less.

Essential oil is another staple to have in your refrigerator at all times since you'll be taking one to two tablespoons daily. There are a number of high-quality brands available and each of these is made from organically grown, cold-pressed nuts and seeds and blended to supply a 1-1 ratio of Omega 3 and Omega 6 essential fatty acids. Omega Nutrition makes a great five-oil blend called Essential Blend while Udo's Choice is another top-quality product designed and marketed by Udo Erasmus, author of Fats That Heal, Fats That Kill.

Omega Nutrition also markets organically grown, cold-pressed hemp seed oil, which has both Omega 3 and 6 fatty acids occurring naturally, in a perfect 1-1 ratio.

All of these oils have a wonderful, nutty flavour and are easy to digest regardless of how you choose to ingest them. Some people will simply pour them into a tablespoon and take one or two a day while others, who object to drinking oil straight from the bottle, like to mix them in with their blender drinks a couple of times a day. It is possible to pour it on warm oatmeal or mix it into salads and other foods but you must be reminded that cold-pressed oils can't be heated above 130 degrees Fahrenheit or the enzymes and nutrients are killed.

Also on the supplements list is soy lecithin granules, which are easy to find at any health food store. You should be able to purchase this in bulk form in almost any size you wish, though often you find it in pre-packaged sizes of 500 grams, one and two kilograms.

Lecithin can also be found in liquid form or in capsules and any way you take it is fine. However, tablet form for any supplement is the least cost-effective method since any time you purchase vitamins, minerals, or any other supplement in tablet or capsule form, you pay more to begin with, plus there is going to be goods and service tax and provincial sales tax on top of the price. Any food product purchased in bulk form, including protein powder, is excluded from these annoying taxes.

Rounding out the list of essential supplements is apple cider vinegar. Again this can be purchased at any health food store and there are a number of excellent brands available all of which are made from organically grown apples and which are neither pasteurized nor filtered. We prefer these varieties, believe me. Apple cider vinegar is also available at some retail grocery chains but be certain you are getting what you think you are buying. Some of these products are nothing more than distilled, white vinegar with apple-cider flavouring. There is a big, big difference so if there is any doubt in your mind, ask questions. Better still, stick to the health food stores.

Vitamin and mineral supplements to have on hand include vitamin C - preferably with bioflavenoids for better absorption - zinc tablets (25 mg or less in strength is recommended) and maybe a B-complex tablet. You shouldn't need a multi-vitamin tablet as long as you are following the nutritional guidelines and are getting enough fresh, raw food in a variety of colours each day in your diet.

Another little item you'll want to have around the house is green tea. The best type - and there are hundreds of varieties and brands on the market in North America - is organically grown Japanese variety. Drink green tea every day to benefit from the rich source of flavenoids and its strong antioxidant qualities.

By the way, I have mentioned the term bioflavenoids a number of times, particularly in conjunction with vitamins such as vitamin C. Biovlavenoids are not vitamins themselves, but are essential to our health because they are known as accessory nutrients. They are sometimes called vitamin P or vitamin K. They are water-soluble nutrients that give many fruits and vegetables their colours. These include grapes, tomatoes, peppers, plums, cabbage, broccoli, prunes, cherries and apricots to name a few. The white part of citrus fruits - between the peel and the flesh, is also full of bioflavenoids.

Bioflavenoids are similar in action to vitamin C in that they strengthen capillaries (small blood vessels) and regulate capillary permeability to prevent allergies, diminish bruising and reduce inflammation. They are also powerful antioxidants, which means they are able to stabilize free radicals.

Appliances: The first thing on your list of items to purchase is a blender - provided you don't already own one, that is. You're going to need one of these since protein shakes will become a daily ritual from now on.

Be sure and choose a good quality one, preferably with a glass carafe as opposed to a plastic one. They tend to stand up to every day use better and they don't absorb odours like the plastic tends to do after a period of daily use.

Also choose a brand such as Osterizer, which allows you to remove the cover and add fruits and other supplements while it is in the process of blending. Otherwise you end up with your protein shake all over the kitchen if you take off the lid while it's in progress.

If you don't own a toaster-oven, this also makes an ideal kitchen companion. This is because it is simpler to bake or broil chicken breasts and other portion-sized cuts of meat and fish in one of these ovens than it is to bake or broil in a conventional oven. The latter uses a lot more energy and produces a lot more heat in the house, especially in summer months when you are trying to keep the heat out and the cool air inside. These little ovens can accommodate as many as four or five single-sized portions like boneless, skinless chicken breasts or salmon steaks and you can eat one immediately, then store the remainder under cellophane in the refrigerator to be microwaved later at work or at home.

Since you will probably be eating rice up to three or more times per week, you might also want to invest in a rice cooker although rice cooks just as easily, and just as fast on top of the stove in a good metal pot with a tight-fitting lid.

The only other expensive item recommended is a juicer for making fresh fruit and vegetable juices. There are plenty on the market, ranging in price from less than $30 to several thousand dollars if you prefer a commercial quality machine.

There are several good ones in the mid-range including the Champion, the Green Machine and, my personal favourite, the L'Equip, which comes with a 12-year guarantee, is easy to clean, and has stainless steel components along with a powerful 3/4 hp electric motor.

The latter is a centrifugal style juicer, which relies on a rapidly spinning basket to grind and extract the juice while extracting the pulp. The former two are grinding or masticating style juicers which extract less juice from the fruits and vegetables than do the centrifugal type, but the juice is of a better quality and is more stable than that produced by the centrifugal types. In fact, juice from the Green Machine can be stored for several days without losing its nutrients to the process of oxidation. On the other hand, juice from centrifugal juicers must be consumed immediately in order to reap the full benefits.

Low-tech kitchen implements to have on hand include a couple of metal whisks - those elongated, bent-wire devices used to whip egg whites and blend things in bowls, a spatula and a few wooden spoons, which come in handy for a lot of reasons, and a good garlic press.

Another handy gadget is a sieve - either metal or plastic, and a strainer. The sieve can be used in a number of ways but you'll likely need a way to strain the pulp out of your carrot juice so this is the handiest item to have on hand for this purpose. A strainer, or even a colander, is also handy to have for draining pasta.

Meanwhile, you might also want to invest in a steam basket so you can steam veggies to just the right degree of doneness. These are usually inexpensive little basket-like items that can fold up like a camera aperture and sit on the bottom of a pot on short legs, above the boiling water, in the steam given off.

Recipes and Meals

Some men like to cook and know their way around a kitchen. For others - most others, it seems - A kitchen is foreign territory. Any man can cook and look after his own nutritional needs regardless of how inept he may think he is in the kitchen. Some also think it's somehow unmanly to do their own cooking or that they might have to get in touch with their feminine side in order to boil rice. Get over it.

Cooking is simple and fun. Once you get the hang of it, and gain a little confidence in your abilities, once the mysteries are overcome, you'll find there was nothing to be afraid of in the first place.

Assuming you've paid some attention to the earlier chapter, which deals with stocking your kitchen, you should have no difficulty putting together these simple meals. Everything outlined here is fundamental nutrition. If you eat nothing else, there are enough recipes here to turn you into rock-hard muscle and a lean, well-defined man.

You may notice that in some cases I'm advocating the use of a spray cooking oil for some purposes. Ordinarily I wouldn't recommend using these types of lubricants, but a one-second spray leaves less than a gram of oil on the surface of the fry pan and only constitutes about six calories.

Be certain, if you are using these spray oils, that you look for the ones which contain olive oil and which use some inert gas as a propellant, rather than butane gas or some kind of CFC gas that

170
will not only be toxic, but will only help to deplete the ozone layer above the earth.

However, if you'd prefer not to use these sprays, by all means use a small pat of butter, a little olive oil, or even just a couple of tablespoons of water to prevent the foods from sticking.

Salads

The best, easiest-to-make salad dressing ever

* 4 ounces (four) cold-pressed, organically grown flax seed oil
* 4 ounces (four) organic, raw, unpasteurised apple cider vinegar
* 1 teaspoon (one) spike

Combine all three ingredients in an eight-ounce glass bottle with a secure, screw-down lid. Place lid on bottle and shake vigorously for 10-20 seconds until all ingredients are well blended.

This dressing tastes so good, everyone who tries it will not only be amazed that you made it yourself, but also will immediately ask you for the recipe. Later you can trade stories about the kids and go shopping together if you'd like. (I'm teasing)

For a tasty variation on this basic dressing recipe, crush a whole clove of fresh, organically grown garlic into the oil and let it sit for 10 or 15 minutes before adding the remaining ingredients.

Keep this dressing in your refrigerator at all times and give it a good shake just before pouring onto your salad.

Dynamite Pasta Salad

* 1 cup (eight ounces) organic, cheese-filled tortellini and/or ravioli (preferably whole-wheat) - preferably the frozen variety
* 1 cup (eight ounces) organic, spiral rotini noodles
* 1/2 cup (four ounces) each of sliced, raw carrots, sliced red and green peppers, sliced snow peas and chopped cauliflower

* 3-4 ounces (three - four) salad dressing
* Two tablespoons finely chopped fresh, organically grown dill weed

Into a large pot of boiling water, add the rotini and the filled pasta and allow it to cook for about five minutes.

Add the carrots and allow them to boil with the pasta for another two minutes, and then add the cauliflower for another minute - but no longer. Everything should only be boiling for a total of eight minutes.

Take everything off the stove and strain pasta, carrot and cauliflower through a sieve or large colander and run everything under ice-cold water for a few minutes to prevent further cooking and to cool the mixture quickly.

Pour all ingredients into a plastic or Tupperware container with a snap-on lid. Add all other vegetables, then add salad dressing and dill weed, place lid on tightly and shake both up and down and side to side for a minute or so to get everything mixed together and well coated with both dressing and dill weed.

You're going to like this stuff so much you may think you've died and gone to heaven - and so will everyone else who tries it. If you don't share it with anyone, this much salad should last about six meals as an accompaniment to your chicken breasts and green salad.

Killer Green Salad with seeds

* 2 cups (about one and a half large handfuls) organically grown, mixed baby greens or organic spring mix.
* 2 tablespoons salad dressing
* 1 tablespoon each of organic, raw pumpkin seeds and organic, raw sunflower seeds
* 1 tablespoon (optional) Italiano cheese (this is a shredded, six-cheese blend of mozzarella, provolone, Parmesan, Romano, fontina and asiago cheeses)

Put everything together in one plastic container with an airtight, snap-on led and shake vigorously until all ingredients are well mixed. Transfer onto a plate and enjoy.

Be forewarned that this creation is so good and so easy, you'll wonder how you've lived this long without discovering such a mega secret of life. Be warned also, that people will follow you, hound you and in general really want to know how you make something that tastes so good, yet is so good for you. Enjoy the feeling.

Mixed Vegetable Salad

* 1 cup (eight-10 ounces) mixture of organically grown carrot sticks, celery sticks, zucchini sticks, sliced red and green bell peppers.
* 1 tablespoon salad dressing
* 1 teaspoon chopped, fresh, organically grown dill weed

Combine everything in the same type of plastic, airtight, snap-on covered plastic container and shake gently a few times so all the veggies are evenly coated with both dressing and dill weed. Pour out of plastic container onto a plate. Serve on the side with chicken breasts, rice and salsa for a satisfying, balanced, nutritional meal.

Breakfast

Breakfast Burritos

* 3-4 (three to four) egg whites
* 1 (one) whole egg
* 1/2 cup sliced or chopped organically grown red and green bell peppers and tomatoes.
* 1 tablespoon (one) basil pesto sauce (see recipe)
* 1 tablespoon (one) Italiano cheese (optional)
* 1 (one) organically grown, whole-wheat flour burrito

Separate egg whites from egg yolks for all but one of the eggs. Do this by cracking the egg on the side of a mixing bowl, splitting it apart and passing the yolk gently back and forth from one half the shell to the other until all the white has fallen into the bowl and only the yolk remains.

Put the whites and the whole egg into the mixing bowl and whisk briskly until there is only an homogenous, well-blended mixture.

Spray vegetable oil spray onto bottom of fry pan and preheat slightly on a medium-low setting. Pour in egg mixture, season well with spike and cover for a few minutes.

Meanwhile, spread basil pesto mixture over surface of burrito.

When omelet mixture has sufficiently firmed up inside the fry pan, sprinkle the grated cheese mix over the surface, return the lid and take off the heat for about 30 seconds - just until it melts).

Using a spatula, or egg-flipper, transfer whole omelet to burrito (it should fit perfectly). Spread the pepper and tomato mixture over half the surface and roll up the burrito as per the instructions on the burrito package. If there are no instructions, just roll it up so you can hold it in one hand and eat it.

These things are so good you'll likely want to eat them occasionally for meals other than breakfast. If you do, go right ahead.

Incidentally, you can occasionally substitute any one of the flavoured burritos they currently have on the market for the whole-wheat one, but there is a lot more fibre in the whole wheat. They have pesto-flavoured burritos, but they don't taste as good as spreading your own pesto on the burrito itself.

Super Oat Bran or Super Oatmeal

* 1/2 cup (four ounces) organically grown oat bran or organically grown oatmeal
* 1 scoop (28-20 grams) ion whey exchange protein powder - any flavour)
* 1 cup (eight-10 ounces) purified or distilled water

Place the water and the oat bran into a small pot on the stove and turn heat to medium high with lid off.

When oat bran begins to boil, turn heat to medium-low and stir occasionally until it begins to thicken. Once it thickens somewhat, remove from heat and cover with lid for two or three

174

minutes to give it time to thicken a little more and to finish cooking.

Remove lid and add protein powder, then stir well until the mixture is well blended.

Pour into a bowl; add a little soy milk, if necessary. Enjoy.

This is an ultra-easy and quick breakfast idea that takes less than 10 minutes from start to finish. It has plenty of fibre and about 25-30 grams of high-quality protein. The oat bran version will have a slightly higher fibre content but both taste equally delicious.

Carrot and apple juice

* 6-8 (six to eight) whole, raw, organically grown carrots with butt-ends cut off about one inch.
* 1 or 2 (one or two) whole, organically grown apples - any variety
* a few sprigs of parsley

Push each of the carrots slowly through your juicer, followed by the apples, then the parsley. Stir the juice a little to completely blend the different flavours, then pour through a sieve to remove some of the fine pulp and fibres that will still be in the juice. You don't have to do this step however, since the pulp tastes wonderful and does a wonderful number on your intestines as it moves through your digestive system first thing in the morning. If you remember to begin each morning, or at least three-to-five mornings a week, with this little number, your body will love you for it, and you'll feel like you're 10 years old again - limber, spry, full of energy, and as pain-free as a school kid.

Entrees

Salsa

* 3 (three) large, ripe tomatoes
* 1/3 cup (one third cup) finely chopped organic onions
* 1/4 cup (one quarter cup) organic, raw, unpasteurized apple cider vinegar
* 1 or 2 (one or two) jalapeno pepper, stemmed and coarsely chopped

* 2 or 3 (two or three) cloves garlic, peeled and coarsely
    chopped
* 2 tablespoons (two) cold-pressed, organic, extra virgin
    olive oil
* 1/2 teaspoon Spike seasoning
* 1/3 cup (one third cup) fresh, organic cilantro

Slice the tomatoes in half and gently squeeze out and discard the seeds and liquid. Cut into chunks. Place all ingredients in a food processor or a blender and process until fairly smooth.

You can vary the amount of garlic and/or jalapeno peppers depending on how hot you like your salsa. If you like, you can double this recipe and make enough to last a few days or a week, depending on how often you are using salsa. It's delicious, nutritious and good for so many things inside your body; you may want to eat it everyday. Go ahead.

Pasta With Basil Pesto Sauce

Pesto Sauce

* 1 cup (eight to 10 ounces) fresh, whole, organically grown
    basil leaves - any variety such as sweet basil, ruby etc.
* 2 cloves (two) fresh, organically grown garlic
* 1/4 cup (two or three ounces) cold-pressed, organically
    grown extra virgin olive oil
* 2 tablespoons (two) raw, organically grown pine nuts
* 1-2 tablespoons (one to two) freshly ground Parmesan
    cheese

Place all ingredients in a blender or food processor and blend for a minute or so until it is a smooth, green paste. If it is too thick, add a little more olive oil as it is blending. You want it to be the consistency of ketchup when it's finished, but not too runny. For the sundried tomato version or the sundried tomato and sundried red pepper versions, simply reconstitute a 1/2 cup organically grown, sundried tomatoes and/or organically grown sundried red peppers in a little fresh, boiling purified water. Let them boil a minute or two, then remove from heat and leave them in the pot, in the water until the water is all drawn up into the tomatoes and peppers.

176

Add these to the pesto mixture while you are processing it.

Pasta

* 3 or 4 ounces (three or four) whole wheat, organic pasta -
    any variety.
* enough fresh, purified or distilled water to boil the pasta.

Cook pasta just until it is firm to the teeth (il dente), drain and place back in pot in which it was boiled. Add a couple tablespoons of the peso sauce and gently stir or shake until it is coated. Enjoy.

Save the leftover peso in an airtight container in the fridge and use it for pasta, chicken recipes and breakfast burritos.

Spiked Chicken Breasts

* any number of fresh, organic (if possible) boneless,
    skinless chicken breasts
* enough spike seasoning to cover them

Spray the top of the broiler pan lightly and evenly with cooking oil spray. Lay the breasts side by side on top of the tray, arranging them so the fat ends and narrow ends are alternated.

Sprinkle Spike seasoning over all the breasts and place in you toaster oven (or regular oven if you have no toaster oven). Bake at 425 degrees for about 20 minutes, or until they look and smell done.

Save leftover breasts on a covered platter in the fridge. They'll keep for three or four days and you can take out one and warm it in a microwave at home or at the office anytime you need a meal.

Cooking chicken doesn't get any simpler or better tasting than this. You'll find the Spike seasoning does a wonderful job of complimenting the flavour of the chicken without being too heavy. Served with rice and salsa or pasta salad and either green salad or a veggie salad, this is a high-protein, low-fat power meal.

Chicken with Sundried Tomato Basil

* any number of chicken breasts
* 1 tablespoon sundried tomato basil pesto or sundried tomato-red pepper basil pesto

Season and bake chicken breasts as per the instructions for Spike chicken breasts. Put on a plate and place a tablespoonful of the pesto sauce on top of the chicken breast and spread it over the entire surface.

This is a wonderful variation on the Spiked chicken breasts. You can enjoy it with each of the three types of basil pesto for a little variation in your chicken breast menu.

Brown Rice With Salsa

* 1 cup (eight to 10 ounces) organic, brown rice - long grain, short grain or brown Basmati
* 2 cups (two) fresh, distilled or purified water
* 3-4 tablespoons (three to four) salsa sauce

Put the rice and water into a medium-sized pot; place tight-fitting lid on and place on high heat. When rice begins to boil, turn heat down to medium low and let it simmer, with lid securely fastened, for about 30 minutes - don't lift lid or stir rice during this time.

When rice is cooked, remove from heat and let sit with lid on so steam can continue cooking the rice a little longer and all the water is drawn up into the grains.

Spoon out rice onto plate and cover generously with salsa sauce. Enjoy.

This is a quick, easy way to spruce up ordinary brown rice. Put salsa sauce on baked potatoes and baked sweet potatoes (yams) too instead of butter or sour cream. It gives it a wonderful flavour and it helps maintain a high metabolic rate.

No-Crust Pizza

* 1/2 cup (one half) coarsely chopped or sliced organically grown zucchini
* 1/2 cup (one half) coarsely chopped or sliced organic, sweet white or red onion
* 1/2 cup (one half) coarsely chopped or sliced organic, red and green bell peppers
* 1/2 cup (one half) coarsely chopped or diced organically grown tomatoes
* 1/2 to 1 whole clove fresh, organically grown garlic - finely chopped or minced
* 1/2 cup grated, organic mozzarella cheese or soy cheese substitute
* Spike seasoning to taste

Spray the bottom of a covered skillet with spray cooking oil and place over medium-low heat. Place all the veggies, including the garlic, in the pan, season lightly with spike and gently sauté them, stirring occasionally, until they are still brightly coloured, but slightly blanched (cooked).

Remove from burner and sprinkle cheese over entire surface of veggies, then replace lid. Leave for a minute or two until the cheese is melted over the veggies, then spoon it out, using a spatula, onto a plate. This recipe will feed two or three people or make a wonderful side dish for your chicken or fish.

Parchment-baked, Herbed Fish

* 1 (one) 6-8-ounce (six-eight-ounce) boneless, skinless filet of fish - salmon, cod, halibut or any other, as long as it is fresh
* chopped fresh, organically grown dill and/or tarragon
* 1 sheet (one) parchment cooking paper

Place fish filet in centre of parchment paper and sprinkle generously with herbs. Sprinkle lightly with Spike seasoning, but this is purely optional. Fold sides of paper over fish and fold up ends so it makes a neat, tightly sealed package. Bake at 300 degrees in your toaster oven for 10-12 minutes (or microwave on high for 5 minutes).

Remove from oven and let sit for a few minutes so fish can continue cooking in steam and its own juices. Cut paper from around fish, but leave the bottom paper under the filet and place on your plate. Serve with any of the above salads, but the fresh veggie salad is preferred. Also serve with rice or baked potato and salsa.

Lunches and Drinks

Chicken-vegetable Pita Pockets

* 1 cold chicken breast, sliced into thin strips
* 1/3 cup sliced, organic mixed vegetables - red and green bell peppers, cucumbers, and tomatoes
* 1 tablespoon basil pesto sauce
* 1 organic, whole-wheat pita pocket

Combine all ingredients in a small mixing bowl and toss with a fork until thoroughly mixed and covered in pesto sauce. Spoon into pita pocket and enjoy with a green salad and a cup of green tea.

Easy Salmon or Tuna Salad

* 1 can (one) sockeye salmon or else whole yellow fin or albacore tuna
* 2 cups (one or two big handfuls) spring mix or mixed baby green, organically grown salad mix
* 1-2 tablespoons salad dressing

Mix salad as per instructions earlier in this chapter and arrange on plate with a hole in the centre for the salmon or tuna. Open the can of fish, drain well and, in the case of the salmon, remove all bones and skin. Place fish in centre of salad and enjoy this healthy, high-protein, high-fibre lunch.

Power Shakes

* 1 cup (eight to 10 ounces) water or fruit juice
* 2 tablespoons (two) soy lecithin granules
* 1 tablespoon (one) essential oils
* 1 scoop (one) ion-exchange whey protein powder - any flavour
* several ice cubes

Place all ingredients, except for the protein powder, in a blender ,and blend at a low speed until all the ice is crushed, then increase speed until mixture is well blended. Take lid off blender while it is operating and add the scoop of protein powder. Adding it after the mixture is blended and moving will prevent it from sticking to the edges of the blender, which can be very annoying and wasteful of good protein powder.

Drink slowly, chewing each mouthful like it were solid food before swallowing. Where fruit juice is indicated, the only kind recommended is freshly made orange juice or apple juice. No frozen fruit juice concentrates, unless it is certified organic and unpasteurized. You can buy organic, unpasteurized apple cider, which will do very nicely if you can find it.

Fruit Smoothies

* 1 cup water or fruit juice
* 2 tablespoons soy lecithin granules
* 1 tablespoon essential oil
* 1/4 cup plain, low-fat, organic yoghourt
* 1/2 cup frozen, organic, fresh-frozen strawberries or blueberries
1 scoop protein powder - any flavour, but vanilla would do nicely

Again, place all ingredients but the protein powder in your blender and blend on low speed until mixed and smooth. Turn up the speed and add the protein powder until it is thoroughly mixed. Ice cubes aren't necessary if the fruit is frozen. If not, add a couple of ice cubes to chill the mixture nicely. Remember to chew it thoroughly before swallowing.

Sample Daily Menus

Day 1

Breakfast: Fresh carrot or apple juice

Super oat bran or super oat meal

Black coffee or green tea

Mid-morning snack: Power shake (purified water or fruit juice, scoop of protein powder, soy lecithin granules and essential oil)

Lunch: Green salad

Chicken pita pocket

Black coffee or green tea

Mid-afternoon snack: Power shake or fruit smoothie (purified water or fruit juice, frozen fruit, lecithin, essential oil, plain yogourt and protein powder)

Post workout snack: Power drink - purified water with scoop of protein powder, creatine monohydrate mixed in

Dinner: Spiked chicken breast

Mixed vegetable salad

Brown rice with salsa

Black coffee or green tea

Evening snack: Piece of fresh fruit - organic apple, peach, pear etc. (stay away from bananas because of their high glycemic index (sugar content)

182

Day 2

Breakfast: Freshly squeezed citrus juice blend- orange, grapefruit, lemon

Breakfast burrito

Black coffee or green tea

Mid-morning snack: Power shake (purified water or fruit juice, scoop of protein powder, soy lecithin granules and essential oil)

Lunch: Piece of fresh fruit - organic apple, pear, peach or something similar. Eat this 15-20 minutes before anything else

Salmon or tuna salad

Black coffee or green tea

Mid-afternoon snack: Power shake or fruit smoothie (purified water or fruit juice, frozen fruit, lecithin, essential oil, plain yogourt and protein powder)

Post workout snack: Power shake - purified water with scoop of protein powder, creatine monohydrate mixed in

Dinner: Spiked chicken breast

Green salad

Basil pesto pasta

Black coffee or green tea

Evening snack: Purified water with scoop of protein powder

Day 3

Breakfast: Fresh carrot and apple juice with ginger root

Super oat bran or oatmeal

Black coffee or green tea

Mid-morning snack: Fruit smoothie

Lunch: Pasta salad

Spiked chicken breast

Black coffee or Green tea

Mid-afternoon snack: Power shake

Post workout snack: Power shake - purified water with scoop of protein powder, creatine monohydrate mixed in

Dinner: Parchment-baked, herbed fish

Green salad

Baked potato with salsa

Black coffee or green tea

Evening snack: Chicken pita pocket

This gives you a general idea of how much you should be eating and when you should be eating it. You can mix and match from the recipes that are contained here and you can add more recipes as you go, as long as they meet the nutritional requirements of your new lifestyle.

Conclusion

If you've gotten this far, you've learned a lot about your body - how it functions, how it operates and how to make it do what you want. The information I've presented here is invaluable and can provide you with a basic knowledge you'll need to live a longer, fuller, more functional and more vital life. It's simple, really. But then, often the solution is more simple than we realize or more obvious than we were expecting. There is no mystery to a good, clean, healthy lifestyle nor is there any rocket science behind training your body to be at your command - physically, mentally and emotionally.

Being physically fit promotes a wonderful sense of personal well-being and confidence. It can provide a source of inspiration to those around you - family members, friends, relatives and co-workers. Wouldn't you rather be known for your impressive physical presence than for the size of your bank account or the kind of automobile you drive? Which actually says more about a man, in your own opinion?

Remember too, this is not one-time, do-it-and-forget-it kind of repair job on your body. This is a new lifestyle and as such you must adopt these principles as the mainstay of your life from now on - incorporate them into your daily life. Like they say, there is no finish line and there is also no point at which you will look at yourself in the mirror and say, "There, I'm finally in shape." No, this is only the beginning of a learning curve that will last until the day you finally die. Learn these lessons well but learn more about everything we've discussed. Make it your mission to keep improving your own diet, training, health and well-being. Try and be the guy that is not just "in pretty good shape for his age", but be the guy who is in great shape for any age!

Learning to take responsibility for our own lives and for our own essential needs is as innately human as eating, sleeping and breathing. Somewhere along the line, many of us have either forgotten how to do this, or have digressed into the area of personal wealth and gain, thinking this is the key to happiness.

However, knowing what foods to eat, what minerals to ingest, what vitamins to swallow as well as knowing how to train our muscles and shape our bodies does not necessarily mean we will live longer. A long life is not the automatic consequence of good health and good habits because there are other variables which control our destiny and which can jump out of nowhere to stare us in the face.

Death arrives every moment of every day on this earth in many forms. Accidents happen and there is a certain unpredictable nature to life that occasionally makes a mockery of even the most physically, mentally and emotionally capable beings.

If I learned anything from the death of friends, acquaintances and immediate family members it's that life is not to be taken for granted. The currency of life is often cheap, and one moment you or anybody you know could be living, breathing, laughing and enjoying the world around us; the next moment, it could all be over.

Still, this kind of philosophy is not a license to live a reckless, careless kind of life in which you indulge of everything and anything that presents itself. Rather, it's a wakeup call for the living - to live in the moment more and to try and leave this world a better place than when we arrived.

If you are one of the millions of middle-aged North American men who are in average to poor condition and whose eating habits and recreational lifestyle is taking a disastrous toll on your body, then take heed of this warning. It's not too late to turn things around - to take advantage of the knowledge and technology that is currently available and which grows at an exponential rate. Use it and become healthy and strong and vibrant. And after you do, teach it to others - especially your children - so that they can grow up with a foundation of good health and well-being, instead of poor eating habits and a preference for a sedentary lifestyle. Whatever derogatory statements I have made here about my father, and about all our fathers in general, they still left the world in decent condition for us and also instilled upon us a work ethic that carried them and the world through much of the 20th century. The mistakes they made in regards to health and nutrition were honest ones for the most part, based on the fact that they were either ill-informed or perhaps completely uninformed about the growth in wisdom surrounding matters of health and well-being. They made their way through life mostly by trial and error and fashioned their grown lives based largely on what had been handed down from generation to generation.

We, on the other hand, have volumes of scientific research and advancement at our fingertips. We have a gift of communication available to us that our fathers never dreamed possible. To be uninformed about anything in the 21st century is both unnecessary and unforgivable.

In other words, there are no excuses anymore. As the generation that has changed the world more than all the previous generations combined, we have also made some huge mistakes along the way. We were right about the concept of peace in the world but we were wrong about drugs. We were right about finding our inner child, nurturing our souls and catering to our imaginations but we have been dead wrong about fast food, stressful lifestyles and the concept of acquiring material wealth at the expense of our moral and physical being. Let's change - for the better!

Now take the lessons that you've learned from these pages and grow - physically and spiritually. Assume a new identity - yourself. Use this material as a foundation, but keep adding to your base of knowledge in future years. Constantly strive to keep up with new developments in nutrition and knowledge of the human anatomy. Stay abreast of the times.

In this century we have already finished drawing the map of human genetic code - something that was only a dream just a few short years ago. It was assumed that this human genome project would take until at least 2005 to complete but science has come in with the done deal a full five years ahead of schedule. Armed with this code, science can soon determine an ideal pattern for life and living for every individual on the face of the planet. This is going to mean huge advancements in the war against degenerative diseases of the mind and body while at the same time will mean equally huge advancements in the regenerative aspects of human beings. This could mean new ideas that will keep all of us alive longer and could conceivably make fitter, more vital bodies from those which were previously broken down and overcome by chronic ailments such as arthritis, diabetes and high blood pressure which affect the elderly in disproportionate numbers.

Still, that doesn't mean we should be sitting around on our collective duffs waiting for someone else to invent a means by which we can extend our lives with no effort on our own part. The human body is perfectly capable of healing itself and of regenerating diseased tissue if only we provide it with the right nutrients, vitamins and enzymes to do the job. We are also capable of maintaining our muscle mass and our strength and flexibility long into our golden years but only if we use our limbs the way they were meant to be used.

At the turn of the century, the average human being in North America had a lifespan of less than 50 years but these days it has been expanded to nearly 80 years - in just one century. Nevertheless, while advancements in antiaging techniques and therapies can help us to live longer, it us purely up to the individual as to the quality of life he wishes to enjoy during that extended period. Do you want to simply live longer or do you want to enjoy life for as long as you can?

We are the generation that never wanted to get old and subsequently have lived our lives as though there really was going to be no tomorrow - no consequence to our careless disregard for the physical act of growing up and growing older. But we are now arriving at that place we never wanted to be. We are becoming our fathers - as much as we never wanted this to happen.

But that doesn't mean to say we can't be better men. Not better than our fathers, but better than we are now. We have changed the world so much but there is still so much we have to change. We have made the world around us better, faster, smarter, more technologically advanced than any time in human history. But we still have time to make one last change - the most important one and, the one we haven't given much thought to until now. Our final legacy in the years we have remaining is to leave mankind in better condition than when we arrived.

After all, do we want to leave this earth knowing that we were largely responsible for bringing to the world the legacy of being able to eat more conveniently? To be able to eat while we drive? To eat while we work? To eat while we talk on our cell phones, sit at our computer keyboards. And do we want to know it was we who have ensured the success of fast food franchises and corporate commercialism in places where children still die in the streets of malnutrition? Where children stitch together the designer garments and playthings to feed a never-ending passion for consumption half a world away, yet can't make enough money to buy the articles they are making?

We are the generation that coined the phrase 'global village,' but the hypocrisy of this is that we don't walk the walk, we only talk the talk.

We must change the way we think in order to change any of this. We can no longer afford to be the "me" generation, it's now necessary to become the "we" generation - to undo as much of the bad as we are able and to replace it with as much good as we possibly can in the time we have left. And the best way to accomplish this is by example. We are the teachers and providers of the world now and it is our responsibility to teach the new generations properly and to give them every opportunity to be better than we are - better than we were.

But we must begin by fixing ourselves, by restoring our health and regenerating the degeneration that has taken place. Sure, we still think like young men, but we no longer look that way. We can, however.

And when we've all learned to be accountable for our lives and our ambitions, let's start to undo the harm we've done the world. Let's remove the toxicity and the unhealthy environment and let's alter this collision course we are on for a chemical Armageddon. Let's make the world a healthier, more organic place in which to live.

Your new life begins now. See you in 50 years.

Bibliography
And Additional Reading

Dembe, Elaine. *Passionate Longevity.* Toronto: MacMillan Canada, 1995

Mindell, Dr. Earl. *What You Should Know About Herbs For Your Health.* Book Margins Incorporated, 1996

Mindell, Dr. Earl. *What You Should Know About Trace Minerals.* Book Margins Incorporated, 1997

Graci, Sam. *The Power of Superfoods.* Scarborough, Ontario: Prentice Hall Canada Incorporated, 1997

Walker, Dr. Norman W. *Fresh Vegetable and Fruit Juices.* Phoenix, Ariz.: O'Sullivan, Woodside & Company, 1978

Erasmus, Udo. *Fats That Heal, Fats That Kill.* Vancouver. Alive Books, 1986.

Rebus, Inc. *Fitness, Health & Nutrition: The Gym Workout - Body Sculpting.* Richmond, Virginia: Time-Life Books, 1988

Airola, Dr. Paavo. *Stop Hair Loss.* Sherwood, Oregon: Health Plus, Publishers, 1996

Krohn, Dr. Jacqueline: Taylor, Frances: Prosser, Jinger. *The Whole Way to Natural Detoxification.* Vancouver: Hartley & Marks, 1996

Taub, Edward A. *Balance Your Body, Balance Your Life*. New York: Kensington Publications Corporation, 1999.

Mindell, Dr. Earl. *Earl Mindell's Anti-Aging Bible*. New York: Simon & Schuster Incorporated, 1996.

Mahoney, David J. *The Longevity Strategy: How To Live To 100*. New York: John Wiley & Sons, Incorporated, 1998.

Ullis, Karlis. *Age Right: Turn Back The Clock With A Proven Personalized Antiaging Program*. New York: Simon & Schuster Incorporated, 1999.

Graci, S. *The Power of Superfoods*. Prentice Hall Canada Inc.

9 781553 691938